CPT
Coding Handbook

1999 EDITION

Rita A. Scichilone

MHSA, RRA, CCS, CCS-P

HEALTH FORUM, INC.
An American Hospital Association Company
Chicago

Printed in the United States of America—4/99

Cover design by Tim Kaage
Design and production coordination by Elm Street Publishing Services, Inc.

ISBN: 1-55648-274-4 (with Answers)   1-55648-275-2 (without Answers)

Item Number: 148188 (with Answers)   148189 (without Answers)

I wish to dedicate the efforts of this work to my professional mentor and good friend, Patricia C. Goebel, MS, RRA. Pat has been my role model and spiritual guide for the HIM profession. Since 1984, when I began to explore health information management opportunities by accepting a position in her department at Jennie Edmundson Memorial Hospital in Council Bluffs, Iowa, she has been my inspiration for meeting any challenge. Many a time Pat has lent a listening ear and provided sound advice to keep me on an exciting career track. I owe many of my professional achievements and success to my good friend and her wide network of associates.

Contents

CHAPTER 8   CPT Modifier Usage   81

About the Author

Rita A. Scichilone is a seasoned health information management professional who began her career in 1971 as a medical office assistant. She holds a Masters Degree in Health Services Administration from St. Joseph's College, Windham, Maine, a Bachelor of Science degree in Health Information Management from College of St. Mary, Omaha, Nebraska, and a diploma in Medical Office Assistant from Southeastern Community College, Burlington, Iowa.

Ms. Scichilone has held a variety of positions in health care organizations, including Director of Health Information, Manager of Clinical Data, Supervisor of Health Data Analysis, and Senior Data Analyst. She has served as an adjunct instructor for HIM academic and continuing education programs and continues to provide educational programs for students and active professionals in many settings. Since 1995 she has been Health Information Management Consultant for Professional Management Midwest, Inc., Omaha, Nebraska. In this position, she provides expertise and consultative assistance to both hospitals and physician organizations. Under her direction, the HIM Consulting division has expanded to include a variety of consultation services including medical record review, compliance assessment and education, and coding support.

Always active within professional organizations and willing to help, Ms. Scichilone has held both state and national offices. As an active member of AHIMA since 1986, she served as Chair of the Task Force and Test Construction Committees for the initial CCS-P certification examination and process. In 1996 she was elected to the Council on Certification and will serve as Chair in 1999. Other AHIMA positions include expert panel appointments for coding and Publications Chair and Editor of *CodeWrite* for the Society for Clinical Coding. She was also elected to the Board of Directors for the Iowa Health Information Management association in the past and remains an active member.

Ms. Scichilone is a regular contributor of articles for *Physician Payment Update,* *Outpatient Reimbursement Management,* and *DRG Advisor,* which are newsletters published by American Health Consultants, Atlanta, Georgia. Her articles have also appeared in the *Journal of the American Health Information Management Association* and in *CodeWrite* and *Advance.* In 1996, she was a contributing author of a chapter in *Health Information Management: A Strategic Resource,* published by W.B. Saunders, Philadelphia, Pennsylvania.

Ms. Scichilone and her husband, Marshall, live in Woodbine, Iowa, and have four grown children and one grandson.

Preface

Physician's Current Procedural Terminology (CPT) is published annually by the American Medical Association and used extensively in the United States for data management and reimbursement purposes by health care providers, payers, and health-related agencies. CPT provides a listing of descriptive terms organized by five-digit numbers to provide a uniform language for communication between health care providers, patients, and third parties that pay for or have interest in clinical data generated by health care services. CPT is currently the most widely accepted nomenclature for the reporting of physician services and outpatient surgery facility services.

CPT was designed for use by physicians but is now also used by health care providers of all types to classify, report, and bill for a variety of health care services. In 1987, its use was mandated by HCFA (Health Care Finance Administration) for hospital outpatient surgeries and services and soon a number of third party insurers were requiring use of this coding system for reimbursement for services covered by health plans and policies.

The purpose of any coding system is to allow a number to communicate a unique health service in place of a narrative description that may represent different things to different people. CPT codes improve communication in the health care industry by facilitation of computer processing of claims for payment and allowing comparison of reimbursement with the procedures performed. Most fee schedules for outpatient reimbursement by third party payers are based on CPT codes, making CPT accuracy in reporting a key issue in optimizing reimbursement for services.

This book is written as a handbook to accompany the use of the CPT manual. It provides additional references such as HCFA mandates and helpful tips not contained within the CPT guidelines. Review exercises are contained at the end of each chapter, to be used for class instruction or for self-assessment for a coding professional seeking continuing education.

How to Use This Handbook

This work is designed to be used in the following ways:

- As a textbook for academic programs in Health Information Management and related disciplines which have curriculum requiring clinical data management or medical billing.
- As a text for inservice training programs for health care providers.
- As a self-study guide for individuals desiring to enhance clinical coding skills or preparing for employment where CPT coding knowledge is required.
- As a reference for general use in the health care industry workplace.

The chapters begin with basic information and background data, continue with the application of CPT in the workplace, and conclude with a discussion of the structure and impact of associated reimbursement systems that use CPT. The handbook includes many additional coding guidelines and rules for CPT modifier usage mandated by third party payers. The final chapters of the book provide a comprehensive assessment for review purposes and a list of resources useful for those interested in additional information about a specialty application of CPT that this book does not address.

CPT changes each year as new techniques become available for diagnosis, management, and treatment of health-related conditions. Reimbursement guidelines that affect CPT use also are dynamic as legislative and administrative rules change. This book was written using the 1998 Edition of CPT and incorporates all reimbursement guidelines and information available through authoritative sources up to October 1, 1998.

Acknowledgments

CPT Coding Handbook reflects the contributions and efforts of many people who work together to make health care a satisfying mission and a rewarding career. The AHA Press editors, Marsha Mildred and Rick Hill, have molded this work into a fine sourcebook for coding education and a solid reference for health care professionals who use CPT. My employer, Professional Management Midwest, Inc., provides me with the opportunities and skills to maintain expertise in the rapidly changing field of coding and reimbursement to serve my clients and the industry. Thank you also to the dedicated professionals from the American Medical Association, American Hospital Association, and American Health Information Management Association who help us make sense of a complicated reimbursement system by development of coding resources for health care providers. All of the persons named above have made this project a reality and deserve my sincere appreciation and recognition.

1 CPT Coding System Structure and Format

Physicians have long used some type of procedural coding system internally or as a requirement for payment. Until the 1970s there were more than 100 different procedural coding systems in use, some distinct according to who was paid for the care, others by geographic region, and still others by personal preference. The disparity and lack of uniformity in coding systems made statistical compilation impossible. It was also difficult for health agencies to make decisions on payment for health care services based on reported codes on claim forms. As more care was reimbursed by third parties and computers were used for data processing, a coding system was needed for efficiency in the health care delivery system.

THE HISTORY OF CPT

CPT was first published by the AMA (American Medical Association) in 1966. Subsequent editions followed in 1970, 1973, and 1977 (Fourth Edition). In 1984, the "4" was dropped from the title and an annual update was instituted to cope with the changes required by the increased use of CPT during the 1980s.

The federal government desired a single system that would allow coordination of services and improve the quality of health care data collection concerning health care services and procedures. HCFA (Health Care Financing Administration) was especially interested in development of a coding system that would allow them to determine the appropriate level of reimbursement for physicians and other health care providers for care rendered to Medicare and Medicaid patients. This push by the government moved CPT to the forefront of coding systems during the last decade, in part due to the significant shift of health care from inpatient services to ambulatory care.

Comparison to ICD-9-CM for Diagnosis Coding and Procedure Coding in Hospitals

The ICD-9-CM system has a Volume III that has been used for coding procedures in hospitals since the early 1970s. HCFA considered combining this system with CPT to form the basis of a new system, but this idea was not feasible. Hospitals generally code ambulatory surgeries in both ICD-9-CM and CPT, while physicians exclusively use CPT for reporting their services. Ancillary procedures such as laboratory, radiology, and various therapy provided by hospitals on an outpatient basis are coded only in CPT since reimbursement is based on CPT. Hospitals and other large health care organizations employ CPT in their computer systems referred to as "Charge Masters." Charge Masters organize services in a database where they are mapped to the appropriate CPT code for billing purposes. Code assignment occurs when the service is ordered, often without human intervention.

The two systems were designed for different reasons, which affects the format and usage of codes. ICD-9-CM, Volume III is a classification system designed for statistical tabulation, and CPT is a nomenclature. A classification system groups procedures into logical categories of a similar nature while a nomenclature serves as a naming system for use of preferred terminology in reporting health care services. Because CPT is a system designed for reimbursement rather than classification, it often includes more than one procedure within a code. For example, the code 43648 includes gastrectomy, partial, proximal, thoracic or abdominal approach including esophagogastrostomy, with vagotomy. In ICD-9-CM Volume III, more than one code is required to fully describe a procedure including a vagotomy (43.5 and 44.00).

> *A classification system groups procedures into logical categories of a similar nature while a nomenclature serves as a naming system for use of preferred terminology in reporting health care services.*

Contemporary CPT Use

CPT emerged as the most logical choice for a reporting system because of its widespread acceptance within the medical community.

HCFA signed a limited copyright agreement with the AMA in 1983 allowing it to use CPT in its entirety as part of the new coding system named HCPCS (HCFA's Common Procedure Coding System). The HCPCS system is a three-level coding system which utilizes CPT as the first level. Level II is an alphanumeric system for selected services and procedures which is national in scope and Level III contains alphanumeric codes for carrier-specific or locally performed services.

EXAMPLES

Level I (CPT) code 55700: Biopsy, prostate, needle or punch, single or multiple, any approach

Level II code G0121: Colorectal cancer screening; colonoscopy on individual not meeting criteria for high risk

Level III code W0166: High-risk Cesarean delivery only, including postpartum care

CPT codes are all numbers while Level II codes begin with alpha characters A through V followed by four numbers and Level III codes begin with W, X, Y, or Z.

Future of CPT

ICD-10-PCS is a procedural coding system developed for release in 1998, but its use for ambulatory or physician service billing will not occur until the year 2000. HCFA has assured health care organizations that CPT will be used through the end of this century for reporting health services paid for by government funds. A fifth edition of CPT is under consideration by the AMA in 1999.

ORGANIZATION OF THE BOOK

CPT is a single volume book which includes an introduction, a tabular list of codes and descriptions organized by sections, four appendices, and an index. Within the tabular list are the seven major sections of the coding system:

- Evaluation and Management (E/M)
- Anesthesia
- Surgery
- Radiology
- Pathology
- Laboratory
- Medicine

The listing of procedures is not limited to use by any specialties or groups, so all CPT codes may be used as appropriate to the physicians or facilities that provide the service described by the code. There are two criteria that must be met before the AMA will consider a code for inclusion in CPT:

There are two criteria that must be met before the AMA will consider a code for inclusion in CPT:
1. It must be commonly performed throughout the country, and
2. It must be consistent with contemporary medical practice.

1. It must be commonly performed throughout the country, and
2. It must be consistent with contemporary medical practice.

This is why some forms of alternative medicine therapy or experimental procedures are not found in CPT.

It is also important to note that inclusion in the CPT code book does not imply that the AMA endorses this procedure, nor that the service is a reimbursable procedure that will be covered by any given health care plan. CPT coding guidelines and reimbursement guidelines do not always intersect perfectly, as third party payers may "bundle" some procedures that may be coded separately, according to CPT rules. For example, if a patient receives an injection of a drug during an office visit, it is appropriate according to CPT rules to assign a code for the E/M service, the administration of the injection, and the supply of the material injected. Medicare, however, "bundles" the administration of the injection code into the office visit and does not allow separate payment for it. Medicare also requires that the drug be reported using HCPCS Level II codes rather than the supply code in CPT, since the HCPCS "J" codes are more specific.

THE RELATIONSHIP OF CPT TO PAYMENT FOR SERVICES

There are also many services that have CPT codes, yet are not covered by Medicare, Medicaid, or other health plans. Whether a service is paid for by a health plan should not affect the data collection and reporting by a health care provider. Keeping track of services provided using CPT codes is an excellent method of business management and failure to capture these services may result in a distorted view of productivity and revenue sources for a provider.

Review Exercises

1. CPT was created, maintained, and copyrighted by
   a. the cooperating parties (AHA, AHIMA, NCHS and HCFA).
   b. the AMA (American Medical Association).
   c. the AHA (American Hospital Association).
   d. HCPCS (HCFA Common Procedure Coding System).

2. Which of the following statements is true?
   a. HCPCS is a component of CPT and is administered by the AMA.
   b. CPT is revised every two years under the direction of the AMA.
   c. CPT comprises Level I of HCPCS and is administered by the AMA.
   d. HCFA revises CPT as part of the HCPCS program each year.

3. The two criteria that a CPT code must meet before the AMA will consider it for inclusion in the manual are that it is
   a. commonly performed and consistent with contemporary medical practice.
   b. reimbursed by Medicare and Medicaid and commonly performed.
   c. endorsed by the AMA and consistent with HCFA guidelines for medical practice.
   d. approved by HCFA and consistent with contemporary medical practice.

4. The purpose of CPT is to provide a _____ _____ for communication among physicians, patients, and third party payers.
   a. payment system
   b. classification system
   c. data resource
   d. uniform language

5. The major difference between ICD-9-CM Volume III and CPT is
   a. physicians use ICD-9-CM Volume III to report services in hospitals.
   b. ICD-9-CM is a classification system, while CPT is a nomenclature.
   c. CPT is a procedure classification system, while ICD-9-CM Volume III is a nomen-clature designed to create a uniform language for reporting services.
   d. hospitals use ICD-9-CM exclusively to report procedural health services.

2 CPT Conventions and Format

CPT codes are formatted in five-digit numeric codes. In some instances additional numbers may be appended to the code as "modifiers." Modifier usage is described in detail in Chapter 8. Six separate sections in the manual contain codes for related services and contain some guidelines that apply within that section. The terminology used in CPT is intended to serve as "stand-alone" descriptions of medical procedures. In order to save space and make CPT descriptions less verbose, indentation is used throughout the tabular listing. When an entry includes one or more indentions, the verbiage up to the semicolon ";" in the preceding entry is also included in the description for the code with an indented description. It will be rare when two codes indented under the same common terminology stem will be assigned together, although there are occasional circumstances that warrant reporting of both codes.

For example, the CPT code for sigmoidoscopy (45330) has seven additional procedure codes indented under it. Normally only one of these procedures is performed at a given patient encounter. In rare circumstances the patient may require a biopsy of one lesion of the sigmoid colon and have a polyp removed from another location. In this situation, two codes, both indented under the main one, are assigned (45331 and 45333).

EXAMPLES OF CPT CODES

52270   Cystourethroscopy, with internal urethrotomy; female

52275   male

The description for code 52275 reads as follows: Cystourethroscopy, with internal urethrotomy: male. Because these codes are "mutually exclusive," meaning only one or the other can be used, they would never be reported together for the same episode or patient.

99201   Office or other outpatient visit for the evaluation and management of a new patient, which requires these three key components:

- a problem focused history;
- a problem focused examination; and
- straightforward medical decision making

or

65091   Evisceration of ocular contents; without implant

The first code is for cognitive services provided by a physician, while the second is a surgical code that reflects performance of surgical therapy to correct a disease state. Hospital use of CPT in these examples reflect facility use for an outpatient visit in the case of 99201 and the use of the facility for the surgery in 65091. When a hospital uses a CPT code for reporting it

continued

reflects different services than when a physician reports the code. Payment for the codes in the hospital situation includes reimbursement for facility costs such as nursing care, supplies, overhead expense, and administration. Payment in the physician's situation includes reimbursement for the actual performance of the service, practice expense (which includes overhead, staffing, and insurance), and malpractice insurance coverage.

BULLETS, TRIANGLES, AND STARS

Within CPT, there are special symbols that assist the coder in code selection. These symbols are referred to as "Editorial Notations." Some versions of the CPT book created for hospital outpatient coding contain additional editorial notations that are not found in the regular version of CPT and may be helpful for hospital coding and billing. Only CPT conventional symbols are discussed here, as other notations will vary with the individual publisher of the books.

Bullets

A bullet comes before the number in the CPT tabular listing along the left margin.

AN EXAMPLE OF A BULLETED CODE IN THE 1998 CPT BOOK IS:

●99234   Observation of inpatient hospital care, for the evaluation and management of a patient including admission and discharge on the same date which requires these three components:

■ a detailed or comprehensive history;
■ a detailed or comprehensive examination; and
■ medical decision making that is straightforward or of low complexity

The bullet beside a CPT code indicates that it is a new code for this particular year. In 1998, CPT added additional codes to report services where admission and discharge occurs on the same calendar date. Physicians would use this code to report inpatient or observation visits to a patient in a hospital bed where admission and discharge occurred on the same calendar date. Hospitals may use this code to report observation (outpatient) services where admission and discharge occur on the same date. Hospital use of this code reports the facility services provided to the patient rather than the cognitive services provided by the physician during a "visit."

The bullet beside a CPT code indicates that it is a new code for this year.

Bullets only appear in the edition of CPT when the code is new. In 1999, the bullets will not appear before the code used in the example above. The purpose of the bullet is to alert health care providers that a new code has been added that may be different from codes available for use in reporting services in the past. In the case of the example given, Initial Observation Care or Initial Hospital Care codes were used even when the admission and discharge both occurred on the same date.

Triangles

The triangle symbol also precedes the code and is found to the left of the code. Triangles also appear for only one year. A triangle is used to indicate that the description of the procedure denoted by the code has been revised for this edition of CPT. Triangles are important because they identify codes that require review to make sure the code

> *A triangle is used to indicate that the description of the procedure denoted by the code has been revised for this edition of CPT.*

selected for a specific procedure is still appropriate. Reimbursement for a procedure may not be correct if the procedure has a revised description that includes or excludes certain conditions. Keeping track of how a code description may have changed from one year to the next is very important for both reimbursement and for data management purposes.

AN EXAMPLE OF A CODE WITH A TRIANGLE FROM
THE 1998 EDITION OF CPT IS:

▲ **31090**   Sinusotomy combined, three or more sinuses (unilateral).

The 1997 edition of CPT for this code shows the description to be "Sinusotomy, combined, three or more sinuses." The word "unilateral" was added in 1998 for clarification to show that this code is a unilateral procedure. Without the addition of the new word "unilateral" the coder may believe that this code is appropriate for a sinustomy performed bilaterally, since the description speaks of three or more. This code is intended for reporting a sinusotomy only on one side of the face.

Stars

Starred procedures, indicated by use of an asterisk following the CPT code, likely have the most impact of all editorial notations on reimbursement. The "star" indicates that the "surgical package" concept (as defined by CPT) does not apply to this code so additional services may be reported. When a surgical procedure is performed there

> *The "star" indicates that the "surgical package" concept (as defined by CPT) does not apply to this code so additional services may be reported.*

are preoperative and postoperative activities that are part of the "package." That is, a surgery code includes preoperative services such as local infiltration, digital block or topical anesthesia, the operation itself, and the normal uncomplicated follow-up care required for the procedure. This is how most third party payers reimburse physicians for surgery—one price for the entire package. The evaluation and management services leading up to the decision to have the surgery are usually not considered part of the package and are coded separately. When a coder does not realize that the "star" indicates the preoperative and postoperative services are not included, there may be services deserving of reimbursement that go unreported. A modifier may be needed on the E/M code to communicate this to the payer by showing that the services are significant, and separately identifiable.

Modifiers communicate additional information when reporting a CPT code. A detailed discussion of modifiers is found in Chapter 8.

HCFA has a slightly different definition of a surgical package which they define as a "global billing package." For Medicare billing the "✱" (or star) has no meaning. Because they are commonly small surgical services often performed in a physician's office that involve a readily identifiable surgical procedure, but include such variable preoperative and postoperative activities, the "package" cannot be applied. There are specific rules in CPT for starred procedures that should be followed when assigning these codes. Additional information is included concerning starred procedures and reimbursement in the Surgery Guidelines in Chapter 7.

AN EXAMPLE OF A STARRED PROCEDURE IN
THE 1999 VERSION OF CPT IS:

20000✱   Incision of soft tissue abscess (e.g., secondary to osteomyelitis),
superficial

The services surrounding this procedure would vary depending on patient condition and/or age and extent of infection, so additional codes would be added on a service-by-service basis in addition to the procedure code of 20000. The code directly underneath this code and indented does not have a star, indicating that normal preoperative and postoperative services are included in the code and no additional codes are assigned to complete the episode.

CPT REVISION AND UPDATE PROCEDURES

CPT codes are owned and copyrighted by the American Medical Association. The effectiveness of CPT as a uniform language for communication between patients, providers, and payers depends upon constant updating to reflect changes in medical practice and to clarify use of codes with controversial reimbursement impact. CPT codes are maintained by the CPT Editorial Panel which is made up of physicians appointed by the AMA and listed in the front of the CPT manual. There is an AMA CPT Advisory Committee made up of physicians from all specialty organizations. A list of members of the Advisory Committee for the current year is also listed at the front of the CPT book. The main objectives of the Advisory Committee are to:

- Serve as a resource to the Editorial Panel by giving advice on procedure coding and nomenclature as relevant to the member's specialty;
- Provide documentation to staff and to the Editorial Panel regarding the medical appropriateness of various medical and surgical procedures, and
- To suggest revisions to CPT.

The Editorial Panel meets each quarter to consider recommendations to revise, update, or modify CPT codes. The AMA requires formal application which includes specific information provided on designated forms and documented with current peer-reviewed literature and data on utilization. Once the Editorial Panel receives a request concerning a code or code(s) one of three actions are possible. The Panel may:

1. Approve the addition of a new code or modification of existing language, in which case the code would appear in a forthcoming edition of CPT;
2. Table an item to obtain further information from additional sources; or
3. Reject an item for inclusion in CPT (see figure 2.1).

FIGURE 2.1   The CPT Process

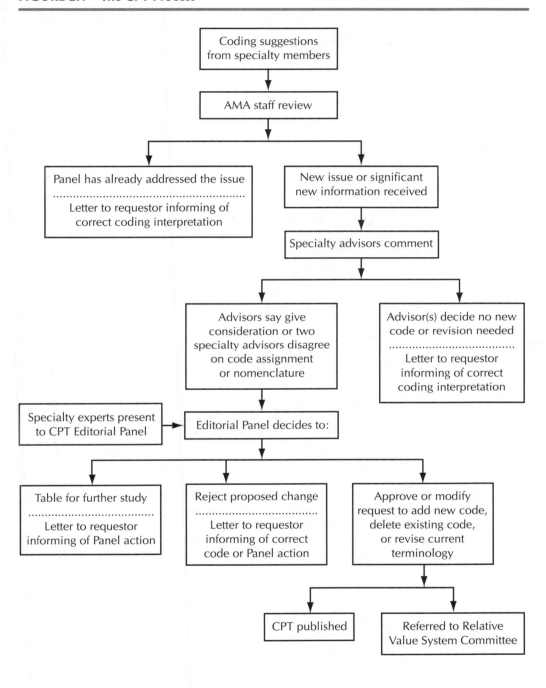

The Panel's decision may be appealed by submitting a written opinion specifically addressing the Panel's stated rationale for the action taken and why it should be not be implemented. An appeal is then referred to the CPT Executive Committee for a decision to reconsider.

Review Exercises

1. Which of the following symbols is used to show that a code description has been revised in the current edition of CPT?
    a. the bullet
    b. the star
    c. the hyphen
    d. the triangle

2. How long do bullets and triangles remain attached to CPT codes?
    a. until the code is revised
    b. three years after publishing
    c. through the current edition year
    d. through the next fiscal year

3. What is the first step in revising a current code or suggesting a new code?
    a. submit a formal written application to HCFA with the details
    b. submit a formal written application to the AMA
    c. petition the Editorial Panel through the Advisory Committees of the AMA
    d. prepare a presentation for the Advisory Committee of the AMA

4. Which CPT symbol has the most effect on reimbursement?
    a. the "✻" (star) because it involves adding additional services that may be reimbursed in addition to the procedure
    b. the "▲"(triangle) because it assists in identifying what is included or excluded in a particular procedure by revising the description
    c. the "●"(bullet) because it assists in pricing new procedures
    d. the indention, since it includes the terminology listed above it up to the semicolon

5. Who can be on the Editorial Panel for CPT Maintenance?
    a. any qualified health care professional with an interest in coding who completes a formal written application and is approved by the American Medical Association
    b. physicians elected by Medical Specialty Societies included in the Advisory Committee listing as published in the front of the CPT book each year
    c. physicians appointed by the American Medical Association
    d. physicians appointed by the Surgeon General of the United States from the list of Advisory Committee members representing each Medical Specialty Society published in the front of the CPT book each year

3 CPT Reporting Requirements

The primary use of CPT coding from a health care provider perspective is to comply with reporting requirements for third party payment or regulatory agencies. Reporting rules for coding may vary slightly depending on the requirements of the entities receiving the information. Because code assignment and reporting of CPT codes are so tightly interwoven, this chapter will explore how CPT is reported and used in current health care delivery systems in the United States.

Although it can be argued that the main purpose of CPT reporting is for reimbursement or payment purposes, it should be understood that data collection facilitated by CPT assignment is also essential for indexing, data analysis, and decision support in health care organizations. This purpose may transcend CPT code assignment for payment when we leave fee-for-service payment and more sophisticated prospective and capitated care systems emerge in health care delivery systems. In these systems the cost of providing services, the complexity of the services, and the outcome of treatments utilizing these services will be more important considerations than the reimbursement amounts attached to each code.

As health care costs have increased, the agencies that pay for care seek new methods of cost control. In the mid 1990s prospective payment systems were introduced by third party payers to limit spending and try to make health care providers more efficient in delivering care. The Resource Based Relative Value Scale (RBRVS) was introduced for physician service reimbursement in 1992. This HCFA-based system provided a systematic method to pay for physician services based on the relative values of physician work, practice expense, and malpractice. For hospital reimbursement, selected payers began to adopt the APG system (Ambulatory Payment Groups). This system employs CPT coding to assign outpatient services to group with a payment value including a "package" of services. At one time the APG system was expected to be adopted by the Medicare program when Congress legislated a prospective payment system be adopted by January 1, 1999.

During 1998, information about the proposed system began to be available. Rather than the APG system, HCFA adopted a modified version called Ambulatory Payment Classifications for use in ambulatory surgical centers and for hospital-based outpatient services. Proposed rules were published for ASC providers June 12, 1998 in the Federal Register (Vol. 63, No. 113 pp. 32290–32521) and for hospitals September 8, 1998 (Vol. 63, No. 173 pp. 47552–47834).

HCFA 1500 AND HCFA 1450 (UB-92) REQUIREMENTS

In the past, health insurance companies had their own forms and these were generally completed and submitted to the payer by the patient. An itemized bill from the physician or hospital was attached, and the payment of benefits was made directly to the patient who, in turn, was responsible for paying the hospital or physician's bill. Now that physicians and hospitals accept assignment of insurance policy benefits and are frequently under contract with health plans, they are often required to complete a claim and file it on behalf of the patient. This establishes a triangular relationship between the three P's of health care delivery: Patient, Provider, and Payer. This triangle replaces the traditional doctor-patient relationship that was typical when patients paid health care costs out-of-pocket and "managed care" discounts and participating agreements were uncommon. The term *provider* is used to describe any purveyor of health services.

Below are some examples of people and facilities referred to as health care providers:

- Hospitals
- Ambulatory surgical centers
- Free-standing radiology centers
- Cancer treatment centers
- Nursing facilities
- Home health agencies
- Durable medical equipment suppliers
- Clinical laboratories
- Physical, occupational, respiratory, and speech therapists
- Nurse practitioners, clinical nurse specialists, and nurse midwives
- Physician assistants
- Physicians and groups of physicians
- Pharmacists
- Clinical social workers and psychologists
- Dialysis centers

Health care providers are required by law to file claims for Medicare patients, whether the claim is assigned or unassigned and whether they participate in the Medicare program or not. The only exception to this rule is for physicians who have "opted out" of the Medicare program and only see Medicare patients through private contracts. This arrangement was made available in 1998.

A physician or hospital is not required to file a claim for a service that is not covered, unless the patient (or his legal representative) insists that the service is covered and wants a formal ruling from HCFA or the health plan involved on the issue. When this happens to a Medicare patient, the provider must file an HCFA claim so that a determination of coverage may be made. As a practical matter, it is recommended that health care providers file claim forms whenever asked to do so by the patient. Official rejection from the insurance company or Medicare may be more readily accepted by a patient than a health care provider's tactful insistence that the patient's services will not be covered by their health plan.

HCFA 1500 Code Reporting

The HCFA 1500 form is a universal Health Insurance Claim Form which is accepted by all general insurance carriers as well as Blue Cross and Blue Shield, CHAMPUS, Medicare, Medicaid, and Medi-Cal. HCFA 1500 forms are printed in red ink so they may be optically scanned by carriers. Only original forms should be used as photocopies are not scannable. The Health Care Financing Administration has indicated to the fiscal intermediaries the blocks on the form that *must* be filled out and the blocks that *may* be filled out. Block 24D is used to report CPT codes to Medicare, CHAMPUS, Medicaid and most other third party payers. The instructions are as follows:

- Enter the procedures, services or supplies using the HCFA common procedure coding system (HCPCS). Multiple modifiers may be required to fully explain the service being reported, but should be continuous. Up to four (two digit) modifiers may be submitted.
- Enter the specific procedure code without a narrative description; however, when an unlisted procedure code is entered, include a narrative description in item 19 if a

coherent description can be given within the confines of that box. Otherwise, an attachment must be submitted with the claim.

When entering an unlisted code, it is always a good idea to attach a copy of the operative or progress notes with the claim so the carrier may price the service appropriately for reimbursement. If there are no modifiers to report on the claim, the space should be left blank, not filled with "00" or any other combination of characters. Failure to use the correct modifiers on a claim may reduce the level of reimbursement, since the carrier would not have complete information about the service provided.

UB-92 Forms for Facility Billing (HCFA 1450)

Hospitals report CPT codes on the HCFA 1450 form, commonly referred to as the UB-92. UB stands for Uniform Bill. It was designed for institutional health care providers because it is suitable for use in billing multiple third party payers. A number of data elements on the form are not required for Medicare billing, but are required for other payers. Reporting of CPT codes is universal, so field locator 44 will be used when there are CPT codes that meet the requirements for reporting.

Health plans may have differing requirements for the reporting of services. For Medicare patients, these are the services that require reporting with a HCPCS (CPT) code:

1. A CPT/HCPCS code is expected whenever revenue code 36X is used indicating operating room services have been used. Revenue codes are found in field location 42 of the HCFA 1450 form. They describe a specific accommodation, ancillary service, or billing calculation related to the services for which payment is requested. The 36 indicates operating room services. The last digit indicated by the "X" above, is as follows:
   360 = General Classification OR Services
   361 = Minor Surgery
   362 = Organ Transplant
   367 = Kidney Transplant
   369 = Other OR Room Services
2. CPT and/or HCPCS codes are also used for reporting ancillary services such as Emergency Room, Radiology, Laboratory services, Physical, Occupational, and Speech Therapies, Cardiovascular procedures, Endoscopies, Respiratory Therapy, Psychotherapy, Durable Medical Equipment, and specified supplies and drugs.

HCFA also requires hospitals to report an Evaluation and Management CPT code to denote a "visit" in a hospital outpatient department. They direct use of 99201 for new patients and 99211 for established patients regardless of the duration or complexity of the visit. The number of visits is reported in the "units" column of the form. Visits with more than one health care professional, or multiple visits with the same health professional that take place during the same session and at a single location within the hospital, constitute a single visit for this purpose. HCFA instructs hospitals not to report this code if the sole reason for the visit was to undergo a laboratory, radiology, or diagnostic test, or a surgical or occupational therapy or speech/language/hearing therapy test. Reporting the various levels of Evaluation and Management coding is acceptable, rather than using just 99201, but this level of detail is not required for facility reporting.

The prospective payment system introduced for reimbursement of outpatient services late in 1998 for Medicare beneficiaries is expected to be implemented after the year 2000. The Ambulatory Payment Classification system has a methodology that requires hospitals to assign Evaluation and Management codes with designated levels. If this method of grouping medical visits is adopted, then the single code to designate a "visit" will not be possible without loss of revenue. Use of the 99201 or 99211 would cause the service to group to the lowest level of payment, rather than the higher level which is deserved under this method.

Physicians must report the actual level of service rendered when reporting E/M services. The HCPCS/CPT codes are reported in field location 44 of the UB-92.

BUNDLING OF CPT CODES

Bundling is defined as the inclusive grouping of codes related to a procedure when submitting a claim to an insurance plan. Some codes, by nature, are included in other codes that describe a more comprehensive service which encompasses the lesser procedure. In reimbursement systems the more comprehensive code is valued at a rate that includes the lesser procedure, so it becomes inappropriate to report both codes for payment. This practice is referred to as "unbundling." Unbundling is essentially the reporting of multiple procedure codes for a group of procedures covered by a single comprehensive code.

Bundling is employed by the Ambulatory Payment Classification system by packaging certain services within each APC group. The APC groups are assigned based on CPT and/or ICD-9-CM coding assignment for the encounter. With the surgical package represented by a certain APC, pharmaceuticals and surgical supplies are bundled or packaged within the group and may not be billed for separate reimbursement. These packaged services are delineated by the revenue codes associated with each one. There are packaged or bundled services for surgery, medical visits, diagnostic services, radiology services, and other APC groups.

NATIONAL CORRECT CODING INITIATIVE IMPACT ON CPT CODE ASSIGNMENTS

Medicare introduced the National Correct Coding Initiative (NCCI) to provide edits within the claims processing system that would detect and prevent payment of improperly coded services. Correct code reporting means reporting a group of procedures with the appropriate comprehensive code rather than "unbundling" procedures into component parts for the purpose of inappropriate, higher reimbursement amounts. There are two types of unbundling:

1. Unintentional unbundling, which results in a health care organization's misunderstanding of coding guidelines and
2. Intentional unbundling, which is used to maximize insurance payments.

An example of unbundling would be reporting codes 58150, 58700, and 58940 for a total abdominal hysterectomy with removal of tubes and ovaries, rather than reporting the comprehensive code 58150 which includes all three services. Reporting the diagnostic portion of an endoscopic code in addition to the surgical portion is a form of unbundling.

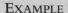

EXAMPLE

Code 43239 is used to report an upper GI endoscopy with a biopsy of the stomach. If code 43235 was assigned for the endoscopy and code 43600 was added for the biopsy this would result in fragmenting services that should use a combination code. Separating a surgical approach from the surgical service is also a form of unbundling. Exploration of the surgical field is included in the CPT code for the surgery reported, so the code for exploratory laparotomy or laparoscopy would not be coded in addition to another surgery performed through the same incision.

The NCCI is revised periodically to reflect HCFA payment policies and coding updates. A variety of sources exist for referencing the current NCCI edits. Many software programs have the edits installed to assist coders in correct coding combinations. Coding references now incorporate NCCI into their products. Written questions about NCCI may be directed to:

HCFA Correct Coding Initiative
AdminaStar Federal
P.O. Box 50469
Indianapolis, IN 46250–0469

STANDARDS OF ETHICAL CPT CODING

Because the codes reported result in payment for services, ethics in coding are important to prevent filing of fraudulent information for the express purpose of obtaining reimbursement for services not rendered, not provided at the level coded, or disguising noncovered services as covered services by manipulation of code assignments on insurance claims. The Oath of Hippocrates, Principles adopted by the American Medical Association (AMA), The American Health Information Management Association (AHIMA), The American Association of Medical Assistants (AAMA), and the National Association of Claims Assistance Professionals, Inc. (NACAP) all speak to standards of conduct which define honorable behavior for health care professionals. Included in these principles are statements concerning coding and reporting of health information.

EXAMPLES OF UNETHICAL OR ILLEGAL CODING:

1. Reporting code numbers or modifiers to increase payment when the documentation or circumstances of the actual service does not warrant it.
2. Coding for procedures that were not performed, or were not performed at the site of service you claim they were.
3. Unbundling services provided into separate codes when a combination or comprehensive code is available for reporting.
4. Failure to code a relevant condition or complication when it is documented in the medical record and meets the requirements for reporting on a standard claim form.
5. Coding services in a manner that makes them "covered" when they are generally "not covered" when reported correctly.
6. Coding another condition as the principal diagnosis or reason for service, when the majority of the patient's treatment is for a preexisting condition that is excluded from reimbursement by the health plan involved.
7. Reporting and billing services as "insurance only," releasing the patient from any obligation to share in the cost of health care services as outlined by the health care plan or provider participation agreement.

EXAMPLES OF ETHICAL CODING

Ethical coding standards in detail may be found in the organizational statements from the organizations listed above. As a general rule, ethical coding includes the following standards of conduct:

1. Anyone responsible for coding is bound to follow published national and state coding guidelines.

continued

2. Codes should be selected and sequenced according to approved guidelines and coding principles, rather than on a basis solely to maximize reimbursement not earned.
3. Codes on a claim form must only be reported when the diagnoses and procedures they represented are documented in the medical record of the patient involved.
4. Health care professionals have an obligation to inform their immediate designated supervisory authority within their organization when they become aware of unethical coding practices at any level. Most organizations have a compliance plan that outlines the process for detection, investigation, and correction of inappropriate coding and billing practices. Ethical coding practices are a key element of any compliance plan.

FALSE CLAIMS ACT AND CPT RELATIONSHIP TO HEALTH CARE FRAUD

Violations of Medicare, Medicaid, and other health insurance plan integrity by a health care provider are usually prosecuted under the False Claims Act. According to the Office of the Inspector General, the most common type of fraud in health care is the filing of false claims or statements that can involve inappropriate CPT codes on claims for payment. The federal False Claims Act governs civil actions for filing false claims. Liability under this law pertains to anyone who knowingly presents or causes to be presented a false or fraudulent claim to the government for payment or approval, or knowingly makes or uses a false record or statement to get a false claim paid or approved by the government.

Penalties for submitting false claims may include criminal prosecution. Civil penalties include treble damages and exclusion from participation in Medicare and/or Medicaid programs. Conviction under this Act makes the person liable to the government for civil penalties of not less than $5,000 and not more than $10,000, plus not less than two and not more than three times the amount per claim that the government sustains as a result of the action.

For physicians, coding professionals, health information managers, and all other health care related personnel, it should be clear that HCPCS/CPT coding carries a significant ethical duty to be used appropriately to report health care services and not used for the purpose of obtaining reimbursement under false pretenses.

The statute of limitations for the False Claims Act is six years. False claims can include health care claims based on services that were not rendered, claims based on false or misleading information (incorrect codes) about the nature of the services rendered, or claims based on false or misleading pricing information. Under this Act a person knowingly engages in misconduct if he or she acted with actual knowledge, reckless disregard, or deliberate ignorance of the information underlying the misconduct.

A False Claims Act case can be initiated by the Department of Justice following an FBI or OIG investigation or a private citizen with information about alleged fraud. This individual files a False Claims Act lawsuit called a Qui Tam or "whistle blower" lawsuit and acts as a "private attorney general" basing the claim on losses suffered by the federal government and the private citizen. After reporting, the Department of Justice investigates the claim for 60 days and decides whether to join in the lawsuit. Once they decide to take the case, the complaint is made public, resulting in negative publicity for the provider.

For physicians, coding professionals, health information managers, and all other health care related personnel, it should be clear that HCPCS/CPT coding carries a significant ethical duty to be used appropriately to report health care services and not used for the purpose of obtaining reimbursement under false pretenses.

Review Exercises

1. The standard claim form for reporting the professional services of physicians and other allied health care professions is the
   a. Uniform Billing-92 (UB-92) Form.
   b. HCFA 1450 Form.
   c. HCFA 1500 Form.
   d. Universal Health Claim Form.

2. Which of the following statements about the reporting of HCPCS/CPT codes is false?
   a. HCPCS/CPT codes are reported only by physicians for professional services claims.
   b. HCPCS/CPT codes have a dual reporting purpose.
   c. HCPCS/CPT codes are reported for facility services as well as professional services.
   d. HCPCS/CPT codes will have an associated revenue code for reporting on insurance claims for facility services.

3. The three P's in a contemporary health care delivery system stand for
   a. Professional Service Providers, Physicians, and Patients.
   b. Providers, Patients, and Payers.
   c. Physicians, Providers, and Patients.
   d. Payers, Physicians, and Patients.

4. The purpose of the National Correct Coding Initiative is to
   a. increase fines and penalties for bundling services into comprehensive CPT codes.
   b. restrict Medicare reimbursement to hospitals for ancillary services.
   c. teach coders how to unbundle codes according to HCFA guidelines.
   d. detect and prevent payment for improperly coded services.

5. A coding consultant is asked to review a physician's coding patterns to evaluate the accuracy and appropriateness of payments. During the course of the review it is discovered that this doctor has been reporting a CPT code for a procedure that he does not even have the equipment to perform. Under the False Claims Act, how far back may he be liable for this fraudulent practice?
   a. 10 years
   b. 6 years
   c. 3 years
   d. 5 years

4 The Medical Record as a Source Document

The source of code validation and the basis for code selection and reporting in CPT is the medical record generated that describes the service reported. Although physicians and/or facilities often designate procedures performed on an encounter form, charge ticket, or billing document, it is the clinical record that is used to validate the level and nature of the services reported by the code.

There are two methods of CPT code assignment. The first is a review of records by a nonphysician coding professional based on record review. The second is assignment of codes based on firsthand or actual knowledge of events (provider assigned coding). Regardless of the method used for code selection (physician selected or non-physician assigned after review of documentation), the clinical record must always support the code assignment. "Manufactured" documentation for the express purpose of supporting a higher level code than the actual service warranted is one method of generating a false claim. This type of documentation may result in substantial fines and penalties and cause loss of privileges or licensure to health care providers. Health care organizations and coding professionals should adopt appropriate methods of identification and prevention of manufactured documentation and avoid any record keeping processes that encourage it.

In hospitals, it is customary for trained coding professionals to select CPT codes based on a review of clinical documentation. Codes are also assigned by a computer program called a Charge Master or Charge Description Master for ancillary services where there is no need for interpretation of clinical data for code selection. Evaluation and Management code selection should be restricted to physician designation, as the medical decision-making component may be difficult to establish by nonphysicians not directly involved in providing the service. Coding professionals and billing personnel may review E/M coding assignments to validate compliance with currently approved coding and documentation guidelines, but code selection without physician input for professional services may result in incorrect code assignment for the actual level of service provided. Facility services may be coded by nonphysicians based on careful review of source documents since medical decision making is not part of coding for institutional services.

USE OF ENCOUNTER FORMS FOR CPT COLLECTION

Within each organization, procedures for communication of the service represented by the CPT code from the patient's interaction with the provider to the insurance claim usually involves the use of an encounter form. This form may also be called the charge ticket, superbill, fee slip, or some other name unique to the organization. One piece of paper shows what was done for the patient (CPT), why it was done (ICD-9-CM/ICD-10), the fee charged, and pertinent demographics of the patient. It often acts as an invoice, receipt, and communication device for health service business management.

Encounter forms may be filled out by hand or computer generated, or a combination of the two may be used. Paperless systems may employ a "virtual" encounter form that is processed electronically until a printed copy is required. Common diagnosis and procedure codes are often part of this form and there is usually space to add additional codes or the information needed to assign additional codes. Managed care plans often use an internal document to record the services rendered to their patients if no HCFA 1500 form is required for payment. This would occur in capitated arrangements.

The danger in overdependence on encounter forms for reporting CPT for reimbursement is the risk that the encounter form and the clinical record tell a different story. This may occur when a physician checks off a procedure code on a form but fails to describe the procedure in the record.

Coding errors are also common if the forms are not reviewed each year for coding changes. An additional concern for CPT reporting accuracy is the limitation of codes required due to physical limitations of a piece of paper. Code reporting should never be restricted to the CPT codes listed on a form, as in many circumstances the range of services provided exceeds the space available.

A mechanism for indicating the sequence or priority of the codes is important, because it may affect the reimbursement. Many insurance plans discount multiple procedures after the primary procedure, so it is important that the highest valued procedure be reported in the first position on a billing document.

Room for including CPT modifiers is also critical for some reporting, as failure to report them may result in denials for reimbursement or claim payment delays for additional review. The practice of using "phantom" codes or service codes that map to CPT codes should be avoided if at all possible, since incorrect mapping can result in incorrect reporting and possible false claims, if a higher payment is obtained than is warranted based on incorrect coding.

Encounter forms should never include provider billing numbers, a check off for "insurance only" payment requests, or any other statement that would facilitate abusive or fraudulent reporting and billing practices. An encounter form is a business office form for communication between the provider, patient, and payer. It is never a substitute for the medical record. Diagnoses must be recorded in the clinical record and all procedures must be described in visit notes or operative reports.

DOCUMENTATION REQUIREMENTS FOR CPT CODE ASSIGNMENTS

Evaluation and Management services have a specific set of documentation requirements that have been approved by HCFA and the AMA for code selection. At the time of development of this handbook, CPT manuals do not include documentation guidelines used by HCFA and/or other third party payers for code selection. In 1998, guidelines developed by HCFA and the AMA in 1995 and 1997 were used to validate E/M code levels. Late in 1998, a "New Framework" document was released for consideration of future changes in an official set of documentation guidelines. The HCFA website (www.hcfa.gov) should be consulted for the latest information concerning current guidelines. It is expected that any guidelines adopted by HCFA would be included in future editions of CPT.

ANALYSIS OF CLINICAL DATA TO IDENTIFY "CODEABLE" PROCEDURES

Transforming records into discrete data elements such as CPT codes on a claim form is no small task. In order to be accurate and complete, skills in interpretation of medical terminology, knowledge of the disease process and treatment methods, and sound application of

CPT coding rules and principles are needed. One systematic method referred to as the "CODER" method of record analysis can assure appropriate analysis of the information resulting in correct coding. It is a five-step process:

1. Case Assessment
2. Overview of Key Reports
3. Data from Clinical Reports
4. Evaluation and Exclusion
5. Review, Refinement, and Reimbursement Impact

Case Assessment is a snapshot view of the case at hand to lay the groundwork for the information needed to code the case. If the service is an outpatient surgery, the coder knows after step 1 that a review of the operative report, pathology report, and all associated services integral to the surgery should be included for comprehensive code assignments for this case. Some services in a hospital or ambulatory surgery center will be Charge Master generated, with the coder adding the procedure codes assigned after review of the medical record data.

Next, an Overview of Key Reports (step 2) is conducted to identify which procedures merit code assignment for the encounter. More than one procedure may be performed at the same session, or the service may include multiple sessions in a series, as in chemotherapy, or physical, occupational, or speech therapy. Key reports in a clinical record include the discharge summary or discharge note, physician orders for related services, history and physical (H & P), progress notes, and operative reports. These are the places where the presence of codeable procedures is found. An overview allows a coder to see what additional information may be needed to code the case.

For example, if a lesion is excised, the CPT code is selected on the basis of size and nature of the lesion. If the size is not recorded on the operative note, it may be found in the H&P, progress notes, or pathology report. If the operative report does not indicate whether the lesion is benign or malignant, the path report is required to assign the correct code. Operative reports have to be read thoroughly so that all procedures performed are coded. Physicians sometimes indicate in the procedure line only the main procedure, and omit secondary procedures that have additional codes assigned. Coders have the responsibility of assigning all components of a procedure without fragmenting the procedure into component parts and "unbundling" when reporting to obtain additional reimbursement not earned.

Step 3, Data from Clinical Reports, identifies associated ancillary codes that should be present, whether they are personally assigned by the coder or physician or selected by Charge Master when the services are ordered. Failure to code all services may result in revenue loss. For prospective payment purposes, selected ancillary services that occur within a "window" of time before surgery are bundled with the surgical payment and are not separately payable to a facility. Knowledge of these requirements is essential for those coding and billing personnel involved with facility reporting of services. For physicians, all services rendered should be captured so that a complete claim for reimbursement is made. Loss of earned revenue occurs when services are provided but not charged to the patient.

Step 4, Evaluation and Exclusion, occurs by the coder examining the codes selected and comparing them to bundling edits or third party payer requirements for grouping codes together under one code. For physician billing of surgery, there is a package of services that includes the preoperative work, the surgery itself, and the normal uncomplicated follow-up care. For many surgical procedures, the approach and/or component procedures are not separately coded or, when a procedure is performed in the office, the "visit" portion of the service may not be separately coded. At this time the code also excludes procedures that are not relevant to the case, since they are part of a more comprehensive procedure already reported.

The last step in HCPCS/CPT code reporting, Review and Refinement, is consideration of the reimbursement impact of code selection and appropriate adjustment and refinement so that all reportable procedures have been included and are sequenced correctly according to payment guidelines appropriate to the situation. For physician services the procedure with the highest RBRVS value (Resource Based Relative Value System) is listed first, followed by procedures with lesser value. This assures that when discounts are applied to multiple procedures in a case the first procedure is paid at full value and the discounts are applied to lesser procedures. Many insurance plans price multiple procedures this way, since the preoperative and postoperative components of the "package" are not duplicated; the procedures after the primary procedure are reduced. Medicare discounts the subsequent procedures by 50 percent from the second up to the fifth procedure. When more than five procedures occur at the same session, submission of documentation and carrier review will determine payment amounts. Other health plans have similar formulas for controlling allowed amounts for multiple procedures performed at the same time or on the same date.

Ambulatory payment grouping or ambulatory payment classification assignments may be affected by the presence or absence of selected codes and the sequencing may affect reimbursement amounts. Therefore, careful attention to coding guidelines is required to assure correct reporting of services.

Case Study and Record Analysis Exercise

Apply the CODER method and analyze the following case for CPT reported procedures.

Chief Complaint: Chest Pain

History and Physical: 12/4/98

Mrs. Patient is a 59-year-old female referred by Dr. Heartwell for diagnostic cardiac evaluation. The patient has known coronary atherosclerotic heart disease with prior anteroseptal myocardial infarction in May of 1998, treated with TPA. Subsequent evaluation with stress echocardiogram study apparently showed no evidence for significant infarction or ongoing ischemia. She has been maintained on medication therapy since that time.

Over the past month, Mrs. Patient has been having increasing symptoms of fatigue and upper left neck discomfort. This occurs usually with activity but most recently has occurred while she is at rest. She was placed on a trial of Ismo a few days ago, but has now developed a significant headache because of it. Because of her known chest and neck pain and the suspicion that she is having increasing symptoms of CAD, she is admitted for cardiac catheterization and possible further intervention.

Admission Medications: Lopressor, 50 mg in the morning, 25 mg at night. Prinivil 20 mg daily, Lasix 20 mg daily, and 1/2 aspirin tablet daily. Takes one Glucophage per day. She denies current tobacco or alcohol use but admits to a history of smoking one pack a day five years ago. She is status post appendectomy and tonsillectomy and had carpal tunnel surgery last June. Allergies include Codeine. Family history is noncontributory. Social history: married with two grown sons. Works in a bakery as a day shift cashier.

ROS: Skin, HEENT, neck, breasts, respiratory negative. Cardiovascular: chest pain complaints of increasing frequency over the last two weeks, history of MI as noted above. Hematologic, GI, GU, Musculoskeletal: No edema reported in extremities. Endocrine, Neurologic, and Psychiatric negative.

Exam

Vital Signs: Stable. Pulse is 64, respiration 16, and B/P is 140/85. Height 5'2" and weight 190 lbs.

General: This is a well-developed, pleasant, and somewhat obese white female in no acute distress; well-oriented to time, place and person; anxious about increased chest pain.

HEENT: Grossly intact. Headaches reported with use of Ismo. Eyes clear, TM and oral mucosa negative. Neck: supple, no decrease in motion, reports pain at times, unremarkable for jugular venous distention or carotid bruits. Thyroid negative. Throat: no redness or exudate, tonsils absent.

Chest: Clear without crackles or wheezes. Respiration unlabored.

Cardiac: Exam reveals soft S1, S2, without murmur or gallop at present. Carotid arteries negative.

Skin: Negative for rashes, ulcers, and scars.

Abdomen: Soft, non-tender, and obese. There is no enlargement of the aorta appreciated. No hepatosplenomegaly appreciated.

Rectal Exam: Grossly heme negative, stool sample obtained for occult blood screening.

Musculoskeletal: Back, spine without kyphosis of scoliosis, normal gait and muscle strength.

Extremities: Femoral arteries and pedal pulses negative. Show 1-2+ distal pulses without edema. No varicosities.

Twelve lead EKG is pending at this time.

Impression: Coronary atherosclerosis history. Signs and symptoms complex of neck discomfort, rule out progressive angina, status post anterior myocardial infarction seven months previous. History of hypertension, slightly elevated today.

Plan: Diagnostic cardiac catheterization for intervention as needed.

John Q. Heartwell, MD
12/4/98 Procedure Note

Preoperative Diagnosis: Unstable angina pectoris, status post inferior myocardial infarction.

Postoperative Diagnosis: Coronary artery disease with symptoms secondary to high-grade circumflex stenosis.

Procedure: Cardiac Catheterization

After informed consent was obtained, the patient was taken to the Cardiac Cath Laboratory where selective angiography of the left and right coronaries was performed, as well as left ventricular cine angiography. Nonionic contrast dye was used. The catheter was removed post procedure with a 6 French sheath left in place in anticipation of possible PTCA intervention. The patient received 1,500 units of heparin prophylactically. A heparin infusion was started for suspected coronary thrombus.

Results:

Hemodynamics: Baseline aortic pressure is 132/83 with a mean of 104 mmHg. Left ventricular pressure is 118/0-10 mmHg. LV pressure post V-gram was 144/10-24 mmHg. Final aortic pressure is 147/85 with a mean of 113 mmHg. There is no significant gradient across the aortic valve.

Left Ventriculography: This demonstrated mild inferior hypokinesis with preserved contractility of remaining wall segments. Calculated ejection fraction was 43 percent. No significant mitral insufficiency was seen.

Coronary Angiography:

   Left Main Coronary Artery: Normal

   Left Anterior Descending Artery: This had a moderate 50–60 percent stenosis in the midportion prior to a distal 2.5 LAD. A 2 mm diagonal branch is present as well.

Circumflex Coronary Artery: This is a large vessel with 99 percent proximal circumflex and a 70–80 percent large obtuse marginal artery branch stenosis. Distal marginal artery was 3 mm in size and wraps the entire lateral wall.

Right Coronary Artery: This is a dominant vessel with a high-grade 90 percent proximal and distal 70 percent narrowing. Somewhat competitive filling of relatively small PDA and LV branches are noted.

Impression: Coronary arteriosclerotic heart disease with symptoms secondary to high-grade circumflex stenosis.

Plan: Options were review regarding possible surgical intervention versus attempted PTCA. Given some degree of prior infarction in the inferior wall making this essentially a single vessel critical disease, attempted intervention with PTCA and possible stenting will be undertaken. If it is unsuccessful, due to the tortuous nature of the obtuse marginal artery, then surgical revascularization may need to be considered to the circumflex, right coronary artery, possible grafting to the CAD, although this admittedly is not critical at this point in time.

John Q. Heartwell, MD

Case Study and Record Analysis Worksheet

1. Case Assessment:

2. Overview of Key Reports:

3. Data from Clinical Reports:

4. Evaluation and Exclusion:

5. Review, Refinement, and Reimbursement Impact:

5 CPT Code Assignment Procedure

After identification of the "codeable" or "reportable" procedures within a medical record or other source document, it is time to explore the steps taken in CPT code assignment. The analysis of the source document and the performance of coding steps occur in tandem to result in a complete database entry or reimbursement claim data set. Omission of any of the steps may result in lack of code specificity and loss of optimal reimbursement. In many health care organizations codes are assigned by shortcut methods using "cheat sheets," encounter forms, or automated methods. If all the steps are not taken the accuracy and data quality of coding cannot be guaranteed.

STEPS IN CODE ASSIGNMENT

The previous chapter addresses the use of the medical record as a source document to gather information required for CPT code assignments. Before any code assignment is attempted, the clinical information must be available to guide the coder.

- **Step 1.** Identify the procedures and services in the encounter by reviewing the source document.
- **Step 2.** Consult the CPT index under the main term for the procedure performed and review any subterms under the main term for the required service.
- **Step 3.** If the term sought is not located under the indexed terms, check the organ or site, condition or eponym, synonym, or abbreviation that describes the procedure or service.
- **Step 4.** Verify the code, codes, or code ranges in the tabular portion of the CPT manual.
- **Step 5.** Read and be guided by any information that may be found in the Notes or Guidelines sections in the appropriate section of CPT or associated with the code(s) in question.
- **Step 6.** Assign the code and verify any specific reporting requirements needed that may affect code selection.

USE OF THE INDEX IN CPT

The CPT book includes a comprehensive index at the back of each manual. The index is the tool used to guide the coder to the appropriate code or range of codes. The main terms in the index appear in boldface type and may have up to three subterms. Main terms can be listed by:

- **Procedure**
  Example: Incision and Drainage
- **Organ or Site**
  Example: Interphalangeal Joint

- **Condition**
  Example: Dislocation

Synonyms, Eponyms, and Abbreviations

A synonym is a term that has the same or similar meaning to another term. An example would be Drill Hole and Craniotomy. An eponym is a term that incorporates a proper name in the term. Two examples might be Bohler Procedure *or* McBurney Operation. Commonly used abbreviations also appear in the CPT index. Examples include D and C, CAT Scan, and MRI.

In the CPT index, the code listings that follow the main term or subterms may be code ranges, a group of codes, or a single code.

EXAMPLE

Cytopathology includes four terms and two subterms, some with code ranges and two with single codes. Any code listed should be checked in the tabular portion of the CPT manual, even if a single code is listed. Because the index only contains a portion of the terminology for the code, a complete review may direct the coder away from this code.

EXAMPLE

The term "Meatoplasty" has a single code list in the index of 69310. In the case of a urologist coding for services, the reporting agency would think it highly unusual that this physician is performing ear surgery. When the tabular portion of CPT is reviewed it becomes evident that this represents a repair of the external auditory canal. When a urologist refers to meatoplasty he is referring to repair of the urethral meatus, better reported by codes such as 53450 or 54360.

Understanding Terminology

Since physicians do not always speak in CPT-compatible language it is critical that non-physicians understand anatomy, physiology, and medical terminology well enough to discern the appropriateness of codes in general. When the terminology is not clear, the physician should be consulted for assistance in finding the right codes.

Two cross references are used in the CPT index. They are "See" and "See Also." The "See" cross reference directs the coder to another term in the index without providing any suggested codes. This often applies to synonyms, eponyms, and abbreviations. In the D and C example above, the index says "See Dilation and Curettage."

EXAMPLE
Drez Procedure

See Incision, Spinal Cord

See also Incision and Drainage

The "See also" directs the coder to another main term for additional information. If the procedure is not listed under the first entry consulted, more information may be found in the cross reference.

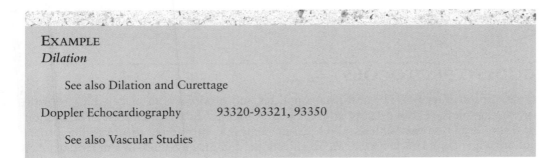

EXAMPLE
Dilation

   See also Dilation and Curettage

Doppler Echocardiography   93320-93321, 93350

   See also Vascular Studies

USE OF NOTES AND GUIDELINES FOUND IN THE CPT MANUAL

CPT contains many notes and special instructions throughout the manual that instruct the coder concerning rules or conditions for code assignment. These notes may have the word "Note" preceding them, they may be enclosed in parentheses, or they may just appear as additional text. Notes may serve to define terms, to direct the coder to another section, or to advise that a code has been deleted and then refer to the new code assignment or the area to look for the same service in the current edition of CPT.

EXAMPLES OF NOTES
Excision, Lesion, Benign

Excision (including simple closure) of benign lesions of skin or subcutaneous tissues (e.g., cicatricial, fibrous, inflammatory, congenital, cystic lesions) including local anesthesia. See appropriate size and area below.

Excision is defined as full-thickness (through the dermis) removal of the following lesions and includes simple (non-layered) closure.

Modifiers

-51 Multiple Procedures: When multiple procedures, other than Evaluation and Management Services, are performed. . . Note: This modifier should not be appended to designated "add-on" codes (e.g., 22585, 22614).

Pathology and Laboratory

80002-80019 have been deleted. To report, see codes under Organ or Disease Oriented Panels.

80040 has been deleted. To report see 80150-80299.

CPT GUIDELINES

Guidelines for use of the CPT coding system are provided at the beginning of each section. All guidelines should be read and understood by coders before attempting to code specific services. The guidelines are section specific, and through the 1998 edition, contain modifiers that are appropriate to use within the section.

CODING PROTOCOLS

Organizations that use CPT must have policies and procedures in place which provide instruction on the entire process from the point of service to the claim form. The portion of this information that addresses code assignments may be referred to as a coding protocol or coding compliance document, organizational coding guidelines, or similar names. A sample exercise is provided to illustrate the usefulness of such a guide to assure correct code assignment for both reimbursement and for data collection and reporting requirements. A coding protocol should include the following:

1. A general policy statement about the commitment of the organization to correct code assignment.
2. The source of the official coding guidelines used that direct code selection.
3. The individuals or persons by job description who are responsible for code selection. It should be clear when physicians select codes, who may change code selection, and by what process.
4. The procedure to follow when the clinical information is not clear enough to assign the correct code.
5. The services performed in the locations that qualify for coding in this protocol.
6. Applicable reporting requirements required by specific agencies.
7. Procedures for correction of inaccurate code assignments in the clinical database and to the agencies where the codes have been reported.

It should be understood that coding protocols are structured around official coding guidelines, but variance between organizations will occur in this process. The sample protocol that follows is not prescriptive of any defined process that must occur for coding, but rather is a representation of how one organization defined the coding process for uniformity of reporting and consistency in coding procedure.

Sample Protocol for ABC Hospitals and Clinics for Emergency Room Coding

Policy Statement:

Evaluation and Management Code Selection for Emergency Room Service Coding

It is the policy of ABC Hospital and Clinic to establish and maintain clinical data coding and billing procedures that promote sound information management and provide appropriate reimbursement for services rendered.

I.   All diagnoses and procedures will be coded using currently accepted ICD-9-CM (ICD-10, when applicable) and CPT guidelines.

   A. The AHA *Coding Clinic for ICD-9-CM* is the only publication recognized as the official source for approved coding guidelines and advice. Therefore this publication will serve as the resource for diagnosis code assignment. For CPT guidance, publication in the AMA publication *CPT Assistant* will serve as an authoritative resource for coding guidance.
   B. The ICD-9-CM code selected will represent the reason(s) for the encounter and other conditions which coexist and affect the management of the patient. Conditions integral to the disease process or conditions that were previously treated but no longer exist should not be coded.
   C. Diagnoses which are documented as "probable," "suspected," "questionable," "rule out," or "working diagnosis" are not to be coded as confirmed diagnoses. Rather, the code for the condition established such as symptoms, signs, abnormal test results, or clinical finding should be used.

II.   Evaluation and Management codes will be selected by the appropriate Emergency Department physician and validated against documentation by the Health Information Management Department at the time of coding for the hospital service.

   A. The physician who signs the Emergency Department medical record is responsible for the selection accuracy of the E/M code assignment for the professional services rendered and reported on the HCFA 1500 form. The same level of code will be used to report the facility fee for the hospital on the HCFA 1450 form. The Medical Record Analyst coding and completing the hospital abstract for the ED case is accountable for making sure the hospital level of visit code matches the physician code selection.
   B. The level of code selected will be in compliance with CPT coding guidelines and current official documentation guidelines published by HCFA and the AMA.
   C. The code level will be verified in accordance with documentation guidelines by the Medical Record Analysts in the HIM Department.
   D. If the documentation supports a higher level of code, then the Medical Record Analyst may change the code assignment when abstracting the case into the hospital information system. This is accomplished by making a notation on the encounter form "Code level adjusted after documentation review." These encounter forms are placed into a special file to be returned to the physician for education concerning level of visit coding.
   E. When the documentation does not support the level of code selected by the physician, the Medical Record Analyst returns the case to the physician for reevaluation and appropriate coding per the HCFA/AMA guidelines. A record of returned cases is

recorded for monthly reporting to the Medical Director of the Emergency Department so that additional education can be made available to the physicians requiring help.

III. When the documentation is unclear concerning the code assignments, the following procedure is followed.

   A. Using the hospital e-mail system, the Medical Record Analyst contacts the ED physician with the Patient Name, Date of ER Service, and the Medical Record Number and states "Coding clarification request: _____." (Concise statement with question clearly indicated.) Name and telephone extension are then included.
   B. The physician will access the documentation on line and respond to the question within 3 working days, either by e-mail or by telephone. If no response is received in 3 days, the Medical Record Analyst should contact the Medical Director of the Emergency Department.
   C. The physician and/or the Medical Director is the final authority concerning code assignment for ED services.
   D. HCFA requirements for reporting the ED "visit" by the hospital are met by assigning codes 99281-99285 according to the code selection by the physician.
   E. The procedures for correction of inaccurate code assignments in the clinical database are as follows:

      1. If the error is discovered within the "7-day bill hold" window, which is 7 days from the date of service, the code may be corrected without further notification, as long as the HIM department and the physician agree on the code choice.
      2. Code changes after the release of the bill should be conducted by completion of a "coding change form" routed through the hospital business office. A copy of this form is attached.

   F. Surgical procedures performed in the Emergency Room will be coded in addition to the Evaluation and Management code for the hospital's services. An Evaluation and Management code will not be reported for physician services if the only service rendered is a surgical procedure such as a laceration repair, where significant Evaluation and Management services were not provided in addition to the procedure.
   G. The only CPT codes appearing on the patient's bill shall reflect actual services rendered in the Emergency Room which are clearly documented in the patient's record.
   H. Procedures will not be unbundled into component parts for the purpose of inappropriate higher reimbursement through payment systems required by third party payers. The National Correct Coding Initiative may be used to determine unbundling, if the CPT manual does not address the circumstances under review.

IV. Coding references are kept current by annual updates to CPT in January and to ICD-9-CM in October. Instruction is provided for both physicians and hospital coding professionals a minimum of twice a year concerning coding and reimbursement issue updates.

Coding Protocol Exercise

1. What required component is missing in ABC's Coding Protocol?

2. Write a paragraph that addresses the missing component that applies to Emergency Department Services.

6 Reimbursement Systems Using CPT

Contemporary reimbursement systems employ CPT coding as a communication tool. CPT codes are readily accepted by computer systems and create a consistent platform for fees and payments when relative value scales are applied. The next sections discuss the health care providers and organizations that utilize CPT as a data collection medium and a mechanism for obtaining payment for services rendered in their billing processes.

PHYSICIAN REIMBURSEMENT

Because CPT is the method used to communicate patient services rendered to third party payers a number of health plans use it as a basis for determining the reimbursement allowed for each service. Managed care organizations contract with physicians for a fee schedule that lists CPT codes with the corresponding amount of payment. Physicians agree when they participate in these plans that they will not expect or require more than this amount in compensation for the patients in the plan. Paying attention to code reporting requirements and bundling of service rules is essential for optimizing reimbursement in a managed care environment or a government-mandated prospective payment system.

There are several methods that physicians use to establish and adjust fees for services. Physician fees in the past were more or less market-driven on what the patient was willing or able to pay. Specialty physicians generally billed higher rates for the same CPT code-reported services such as office visits. Now that many patients do not pay directly for care, the payers for care have a bigger influence on what can be billed for a specific service designated by a CPT code.

The legal methods physicians used in the past to establish fees included use of the Medicare Fee Schedule Amounts; Usual, Customary and Reasonable Amounts per an insurer; Relative Value Studies; Physician Surveys and Published Lists; and other more arbitrary methods such as flat percentage increases each year based on inflation or overhead cost increases. Each of these methods had advantages and disadvantages in keeping fees up-to-date and appropriate.

All major insurance carriers and managed care providers now use either RBRVS or McGraw-Hill relative value scales to monitor a medical practice's charge profile. Therefore these two systems are often referred to as "industry standard" methods for fee structures.

RVS SYSTEMS

Some health plans, including Medicaid in some states, use an RVU (Relative Value Unit) or RVS (Relative Value Scale). McGraw-Hill's *Relative Values for Physicians* has been used since 1984 and reflects medical practice and reimbursement issues through national physician surveys. A relative value unit (RVU) is established for each CPT code so that when a physician creates a fee schedule using this system all fees remain in relationship to each other from the least valued to the most valued. A conversion factor is a multiplier that converts the relative value unit to actual dollar amounts for the fee. In an RVU system, a separate conversion factor is used for each section of CPT since each section represents a different set of physician services.

The procedure for calculating conversion factors is to select 20–30 common procedures from a physician practice and verify CPT code assignments associated with current fees. Using the most recent edition of the McGraw-Hill Relative Value Study, the RVUs are obtained for each of these CPT codes. Each substantive section of codes will require a different conversion factor. These sections are: Anesthesia, Surgery, Radiology, Pathology, Medicine, Evaluation and Management, and HCPCS Level II codes.

The RVUs and the fees are each totaled for the selected procedures. The total fees are divided by the total RVUs to arrive at the conversion factor. This conversion factor is then adjusted to so that the resulting fees are appropriate to the market and the reimbursement potential for the practice location.

RBRVS (RESOURCE BASED RELATIVE VALUE SYSTEM)

The RBRVS system was developed by HCFA and implemented for physician reimbursement for Medicare patients in 1992. RBRVS has now also been adopted by other third party payers in addition to Medicare. The RBRVS philosophy measures the complexity of all services against a commonly performed basic service, such as an office visit. A service that is deemed twice as difficult to perform as this basic service would have a relative value two times the basic value.

The Medicare RBRVS fee schedule is not complete, since all CPT codes are not covered procedures by Medicare, and thus would not have RBRVS values. McGraw-Hill (*The Complete RBRVS*) and perhaps other publishers have used the RBRVS methodology to create values for missing procedures so that it may be used with CPT codes to establish fees and/or reimbursement amounts.

HCFA releases the RBRVS values late each year in a November or December issue of the Federal Register. The Relative Value Units for CPT codes are available on the internet at www.access.gpo.su_docs.

RBRVS used three components to establish value for physician services: Work, Practice Expense, and Malpractice Liability Expense. These elements are adjusted for geographic practice location by applying a GPCI (Geographic Practice Cost Indices) factor to each one. This index is a listing of the specific Medicare localities (by Medicare Carrier Number). There is a GPCI factor for each element. This list is also published in the Federal Register with the fee schedule each year. In 1997 and 1998 Medicare applied a work adjustment factor to manipulate the Medicare fee schedule for budget neutrality without the actual work RVUs for other payers that use RBRVS as a basis for reimbursement. In 1998, that factor was .917. No adjustment factor is applied in FY 1999 for Medicare.

Each of these elements has a value associated with it. To calculate a Medicare fee using RBRVS, use the following formula:

A = Physician Work RVU

B = Practice Expense RVU (Facility or Non-facility as appropriate)

C = Malpractice RVU

A × Work Adjustment Factor (if applicable) × Work GPCI = GPCI Adjusted Work RVU

B × Work Adjustment Factor (if applicable) × Practice Expense GPCI = GPCI Adjusted Practice Expense RVU

C × Work Adjustment Factor (if applicable) × Malpractice GPCI = GPCI Adjusted Malpractice RVU

Add the adjusted RVU components obtained above and round to the fourth decimal point. Then multiply the total geographically adjusted RVU by the appropriate conversion factor. The Medicare conversion factor for 1998 was 36.6873 and applied to all CPT codes in the Medicare fee schedule. Other payers may use conversion factors that apply only to a selected section of CPT, so medical and surgical services may be calculated at different conversion rates. When physicians use the RBRVS method for constructing a fee schedule, often conversion factors are used specific to the range of codes in a certain section of CPT. For example, office visits may be based on one conversion factor while surgical services are based on another, in order to fit the market and the reimbursement allowances for the practice.

Physicians who do not participate in the Medicare program are subject to a limiting charge amount. To calculate that amount using the RBRVS system, the following formula is used:

- **Step 1.** Calculate the participating amount using the method described.
- **Step 2.** Multiply this amount by .95 since nonparticipating physicians receive only 95 percent of the Medicare fee schedule amounts from Medicare. The balance of the charge is assumed by the patient.
- **Step 3.** Compute 115 percent of this amount to reveal the maximum amount that may be charged to a Medicare patient for a particular CPT code representing a service.

EXAMPLE

The participating physician fee amount for code 27130 (total hip replacement) in Medicare location 00 (Nevada) was $1,675.47 in 1998. The physician receives 80 percent of that amount and the patient is responsible for the remaining 20 percent, plus any unmet deductible amounts.

Taking 95 percent of this amount results in a nonparticipating fee of $1,591.70. When this amount is increased to 115 percent, a reimbursement amount of $ 1,830.46 is obtained. This means a nonparticipating physician operating in Nevada could not charge more than $1,830.46 to perform a total hip replacement on a Medicare patient. He or she will receive 80 percent of $1,591.70 from Medicare in payment if they accept assignment. The balance is the responsibility of the patient.

If this physician participated in the Medicare program, the physician would receive $1,675.47 from Medicare.

ASC MEDICARE REIMBURSEMENT

Before 1980, Medicare law limited reimbursement for surgery performed outside the hospital setting. Medicare coverage and reimbursement were not permitted for facility services. Medicare limited reimbursement to 80 percent of physician services in Ambulatory Surgery Centers.

The Omnibus Budget Reconciliation Action (OBRA of 1980) amended the law by allowing a prospective reimbursement amount for facility services furnished in connection with selected procedures. Each year Medicare publishes a list of CPT codes. Under the ASC system, each procedure falls into a designated payment group. In 1998 there were eight groups. One of the major criteria that places a particular CPT code on the list of covered procedures is that it often may be performed on an inpatient basis, but can be performed safely, consistent with accepted medical practice parameters, on an outpatient basis in an ambulatory care setting. Any procedure that can be safely performed in a physician's office without the more sophisticated equipment and conditions found in an ASC are excluded from ASC payment and physician payment would be provided from the Medicare fee schedule. No facility payment would be paid for these procedures.

After the year 2000, Medicare is moving to a prospective payment system based on CPT codes that groups patients into Ambulatory Payment Classification groups for reimbursement. Instead of the eight groups used in the ASC method, the list of ASC covered procedures will expand from the 2,280 CPT codes in 1998 to 2,499 procedures in 1999 and the number of surgical APC groups will increase to 105. New payment rates will be associated with the new APC groups and reimbursement for services in freestanding ASC facilities and hospital outpatient departments will become more similar. It is expected that the APCs for ASC and hospital outpatient procedures will be the same, although the reimbursement allowed may differ by type of facility, at least at the beginning of the PPS implementation.

Freestanding ASC Reimbursement from HCFA

ASCs that are not under the common licensure, governance, and professional supervision of the hospital (i.e., freestanding ASCs) receive 80 percent of a designated labor market-adjusted ASC payment rate. The remaining 20 percent is the patient's responsibility subject to coinsurance and Part B deductible requirements.

Hospital-Based ASC Reimbursement

Section 9343(a) of OBRA 1986 created a new payment method for certain ambulatory surgeries performed on an outpatient basis by hospitals. This prompted the requirement that hospitals report the HCPCS (CPT) codes effective July 1, 1987. For cost reporting periods after October 1, 1987, payment for the covered ASC procedures performed in hospitals is based in part on what Medicare would pay for the procedure if it were performed in a freestanding ASC in the same geographic location as the hospital. Hospitals received a blended amount of the ASC group rate and its reasonable cost. This is predicted to change in the year 2000.

The Balanced Budget Act of 1997 requires implementation of a prospective payment system for Medicare patients that does not use any cost-based amounts. This system categorizes outpatient services into Ambulatory Payment Classifications or APC groups. This new APC system comprises more than 105 groups which replace the current eight groups available in the ASC methodology.

The APC system will cover all aspects of hospital outpatient services that are not already part of a fee schedule or prospectively determined reimbursement amount. This includes surgery, medical visits to the emergency room and hospital clinics, radiology and other diagnostic procedures, and observation room and partial hospitalization services. Not included are rehabilitation procedures like physical, occupational and speech therapy, end stage renal disease services, lab services paid under the clinical laboratory fee schedule, durable medical equipment, and services provided to skilled nursing facility inpatients who are covered by Part A Medicare reimbursement.

Reimbursement will be determined by a relative weight for each APC group which will be wage-adjusted depending on the location of the hospital.

OTHER SYSTEMS

There have been several other reimbursement methods developed that use CPT codes, but none is widely used at this time.

Ambulatory Payment Groups (APGs) have been used by some third party payers including Blue Cross and Blue Shield plans and state Medicaid agencies. APGs use CPT codes to place procedures in specified groups with an assigned relative weight.

Exercises in Reimbursement Optimization Using CPT

1. In the 1998 listing of the Medicare Physician Fee Schedule the following values are listed for code 99284:

   Physician work RVUs   1.95
   Practice expense RVUs   .7
   Malpractice RVUs   .6

   The work adjustment factor applied by Medicare is .917 and the Geographic Practice Cost Indices for Chicago, Illinois where the physician practices are:

   Physician work GPCI   1.028
   Practice expense GPCI   1.084
   Malpractice expense GPCI   1.538

   The 1998 conversion factor designated by Medicare is $36.6873

   What reimbursement can a physician from Chicago expect from Medicare for a Level IV Emergency Department service reported using 99284 (round to nearest dollar)?
   a. $133
   b. $135
   c. $129
   d. $119

2. What is the most significant financial change in Medicare reimbursement that will occur with the adoption of APCs for hospital outpatients?
   a. It replaces ASC payment methodology for outpatient surgery.
   b. It excludes services already paid by fee schedule or other prospective payment methods.
   c. It uses relative values for CPT codes to calculate payments.
   d. It eliminates cost-based reimbursement by hospitals for outpatient services.

The information following is taken from Addendum B from the proposed rules for the APC system in hospital outpatient departments. A nursing home patient is having outpatient surgery for a pressure sore.

3. How many APC groups are available on this page for removal of pressure sores?
   a. 2
   b. 16
   c. 75
   d. 1

4. Which APC group for removal of pressure sores results in the highest reimbursement?
   a. APC 163 (Level III excision/biopsy)
   b. APC 151 (Level I debridement/destruction)
   c. APC 184 (Level IV skin repair)
   d. All APCS have equal reimbursement potential on this page.

5. The proposed rules include a provision to determine the coinsurance that a hospital will collect for a specified APC. Using Addendum B, what is the minimum adjusted coinsurance a hospital could use for a removal of tail bone ulcer described by assignment of CPT code 15922?
   a. $113.03
   b. $396.40
   c. $565.14
   d. $160.43

7 CPT Coding Guidelines

All AMA guidelines for the use of CPT are generally found within the CPT manual in the following locations: *Introduction, Guidelines* preceding each section, *Notes* found under subsection titles, and additional information enclosed in parentheses within code descriptions. The guidelines described in this chapter have been gathered from a variety of third party payer reporting directives, including the National Correct Coding Initiative. Effective coding is accomplished by a synthesis of both resources—payer directives and official guidelines, so that appropriate reimbursement is obtained while preserving data quality and uniformity in reporting. Selected guidelines are reproduced here, but it should be noted that not all guidelines are discussed. Therefore, it is critical that a complete review of the manual be undertaken along with study of these guidelines for comprehensive knowledge of CPT coding rules and payer applications.

EVALUATION AND MANAGEMENT SERVICES

In 1992, new codes were created for reporting visit services performed by physicians. In 1994, HCFA and the AMA collaborated to create a set of documentation guidelines that provided additional criteria and also outlined record requirements for the various levels of service possible to report in this section. In 1997, revised guidelines were released which contained additional documentation requirements for general multi-system and single speciality exams for 10 physician specialty areas. These guidelines became controversial in the physician community and were not implemented in 1998 as planned. The 1998 and 1999 versions of CPT do not contain these guidelines.

Because reimbursement for services is often based on the relative values assigned to these CPT codes by payers, it is essential to consider the documentation guidelines applied in prepayment or postpayment audits by insurers when these codes are assigned.

Evaluation and Management Codes Assignment

Evaluation and Management (E/M) services are generally selected by the provider rendering the care. This process assures that the level of service rendered matches the documentation available and the resulting code results in the appropriate reimbursement. Coding of physician services may be delegated to coding professionals who assign codes based on clinical

> When E/M codes are assigned by non-clinicians, a process must be in place to compare actual services rendered with services documented and appropriate feedback must be given concerning compliance with guidelines in place.

information present in the record. Because E/M services involve medical decision making, delegation of level of service coding should be done with care and only performed by coding professionals who possess the required knowledge level and skills. When E/M codes are assigned by non-clinicians, a process must be in place to compare actual services rendered with services documented and appropriate feedback must be given concerning compliance with guidelines in place.

Hospitals use Evaluation and Management codes for a different purpose. HCFA requires hospitals to report "visit" codes to indicate an encounter in a hospital outpatient department such as a hospital-sponsored clinic or the emergency room. A "visit" is defined as direct personal contact between a registered hospital outpatient and a physician or other person who is authorized by state licensure law and, where applicable, by hospital staff bylaws to order or provide services for the patient for purposes of diagnosis or treatment.

Hospital use of Level I codes

Until prospective payment systems for outpatients are introduced which affect the amount of reimbursement allowed for medical visits, hospitals often use 99201 for new patients and 99211 for established patients, regardless of the duration or complexity of the visit. Because CPT is used in this instance for facility services rather than professional services, the levels of care did not apply in a cost- or charge-based system for payment. Visits with more than one health care professional during the same session and/or at a single location within the hospital constitute a single visit. Services that are provided in addition to the visit, such as laboratory, radiology, diagnostic tests, or other procedures, are coded separately. A CPT E/M code should not be reported if the sole reason for the visit was to undergo ancillary testing without a clinical examination. HCFA instructions before prospective payment was implemented stated that hospitals could report codes 99202-99215, 99281-99288, 92002-92014, or 95105 in lieu of 99201, if they wanted to, but that level of detail was not required. Some hospitals have a fee structure for emergency room charges which uses the five levels of care available for physician services. When the ED physician selects a Level IV code (99284) the hospital also reports this code with charges that reflect facility resource usage for that type of patient. In this system, the ED physician coding drives the hospital facility charge. In the APC system of reimbursement, five levels of coding may result in three levels of reimbursement with the lowest levels (I and II) and the highest levels (III and IV) being combined within an APC group. At the time of this writing, it is not known what guidelines or criteria might be used to determine the levels of codes for facility payments.

Evaluation and Management Code Format

The basic format of E/M services consists of five elements which remain the same for most of the categories:

1. E/M services are comprised of a five-digit unique code number beginning with the first two digits "99."
2. E/M service codes generally identify the place or type of service such as "Initial Hospital Care" or "Emergency Department Services."
3. E/M codes define the extent or level of the professional service such as "detailed history, detailed examination, and medical decision making of moderate complexity."
4. E/M services describe the nature of the presenting problem such as "moderate severity."
5. E/M services have a typical time required to provide a service, although at present, time drives the code selection only in situations where counseling and coordination of care dominate the visit.

New Versus Established Patients

Some CPT code ranges differentiate between new and established patients. The CPT defines a new patient as one who has not received any professional services from a physician or another physician of the same specialty belonging to the same group practice within the past three years. Established patients are those patients who have received services under the same conditions. Location of the practice does not affect this rule. If a patient has received services from a physician before, even if that physician practiced in a different location for the previous visit, he or she would be considered an established patient for reporting purposes. If a physician is new to a group practice but the patient has received services previously from a partner in the group (within the three-year period in the same specialty), the established code is reported, since the patient is not new to the group. New patient codes have a higher RVU assigned due to the extra physician work (obtaining initial history and exam) and the extra practice expense of creating a record, etc. It is important for physicians not to overlook the three-year rule and report new patient codes for those patients who have not been seen in the three-year time frame. Significant revenue loss may occur when this is not monitored.

Coding professionals must obtain and apply the most recent documentation guidelines available by third party payers using CPT E/M codes for reimbursement. Versions of CPT published after the year 2000 may have these guidelines incorporated into the manual.

ANESTHESIA GUIDELINES

Proper reporting of the CPT codes for anesthesia services depends on the insurance carrier involved. Anesthesia services covered in the Medicare program are reported using CPT codes from the anesthesia section of CPT. For many other carriers, anesthesia services are reported using the same codes that the surgeon uses from the Surgery section of CPT that describe the major surgical procedure. Anesthesia services are reported by anesthesiologists, certified registered nurse anesthetists, or other physicians administering anesthesia. Anesthesia services may include general, regional, supplementation of local anesthesia, or other supportive services.

Anesthesia services include the usual preoperative and postoperative visits, the anesthesia care during the procedure, the administration of fluids and/or blood products incident to the anesthesia or the surgery performed, and routine monitoring procedures. Unusual forms of monitoring such as intra-arterial lines, central venous lines, and Swan-Ganz catheterization are not included and should be coded and reported in addition to the anesthesia code.

Anesthesia Sections

The Anesthesia section in CPT is divided into 17 subsections which comprise the following body areas:

- Head
- Neck
- Thorax (Chest Wall and Shoulder Girdle)
- Intrathoracic
- Spine and Spinal Cord
- Upper Abdomen

- Lower Abdomen
- Perineum
- Pelvis (Except Hip)
- Upper Leg (Except Knee)
- Knee and Popliteal Area
- Lower Leg (Below Knee)
- Shoulder and Axilla
- Upper Arm and Elbow
- Forearm, Wrist, and Hand
- Radiological Procedures
- Other Procedures

Resource publications are available that provide a crosswalk of CPT surgical codes to the Anesthesia section such as *1998 Coder's Desk Reference* (Medicode, 1998). Also, the *Relative Value Guide: A Guide for Anesthesia Values* is published each year by the American Society of Anesthesiologists. This resource lists each CPT code applicable to Anesthesia with the base units recommended for each procedure. Anesthesia values are determined by adding this basic value, which is related to the complexity of the service, plus modifying units (if any), plus time units.

Time reporting for anesthesia begins when the anesthesiologist begins to prepare the patient for induction of anesthesia in the operating room or equivalent area and ends when the anesthesiologist or anesthetist is no longer in personal attendance and the patient may be safely placed under postoperative supervision.

For Medicare patients, anesthesia services are paid under the Medicare physician fee schedule. However, instead of relative value units (RVUs), payment for anesthesia is based on the anesthesia relative value guide (RVG) with adjustments made to the conversion factor to ensure payments are consistent with other services which Medicare believes to be comparable in value. Geographic adjustments are made to the conversion factor to allow for location variances. The payment is calculated using the anesthesia relative value with base units per procedure and then 15-minute "actual time" units for both personally performed and medically directed services.

When reporting anesthesia services to Medicare carriers, the elapsed time in minutes is entered on the HCFA 1500 form. All hours are converted to minutes and the total minutes required for the procedure are listed. Minutes should not be rounded up, since extra minutes may begin to overlap in time, especially when anesthesiologists are involved in concurrent procedures.

For Medicare reporting anesthesia may be:

1. **Personally Performed.** Full Medicare reimbursement for allowed amounts is available to anesthesia providers who personally perform anesthesia services alone.

2. **Under Medical Direction.** Medical direction services are billable to Medicare when an anesthesiologist supervises certified registered nurse anesthetists (CRNAs), anesthesia assistants (AAs) or other qualified people in two, three, or four concurrent procedures. In those cases, the payment is split with the CRNA or the AA who was involved in the case. The total reimbursement will not exceed the amount for a solo anesthesiologist practicing in the same location. If it is medically necessary that both a CRNA or an AA and an anesthesiologist be attending the patient, full payment for both providers is available. The anesthesiologist is reimbursed at the personally performed rate, and the CRNA or AA is reimbursed at the non-medically directed rate. HCPCS Level II modifiers are needed to report this situation accurately as CPT does not provide specific modifiers for this purpose. Medical direction is covered by Medicare when the physician does all of the following:

- performs a preanesthesia examination and evaluation
- prescribes an anesthesia plan
- personally participates in the most demanding procedures of the anesthesia plan, including induction and emergence
- ensures that any procedures in the anesthesia plan are performed by a qualified anesthetist
- monitors the course of anesthesia administration at intervals
- remains physically present and available for immediate diagnosis and treatment of emergencies
- provides indicated postanesthesia care

3. **In Teaching Situations.** Special rules exist for an anesthesiologist who is supervising a resident performing a procedure on a Medicare beneficiary. The teaching physician must be present during induction, emergence, and any other portion of the procedure. This is payable on a time basis.

    Documentation within the medical records must indicate the physical presence of the teaching anesthesiologist and participation in the service. The teaching physician is not required to be present during preoperative or postoperative visits.

CRNAs may not report multiple anesthesia services for patients at the same time. Problems often occur when large numbers of short procedures are performed. It would be easy for a CRNA working on cataract surgeries from 8:00 A.M. to noon to report more than four hours of time units, without strict attention to time and never "rounding up" minutes. Total time units cannot ever exceed the amount of time on the clock between the beginning and the end of the service.

For additional information about Medicare billing rules for anesthesia see the *Medicare Carriers Manual Section 15018*. There are selected codes that are bundled into the basic anesthesia fee for Medicare patients and should not be separately billed, except in special circumstances.

These codes, effective with the National Correct Coding Policy in 1998, are:

31500	90835
31505	91000
31515	91055
31527	91105
31622	92511-92533
31645	92543
31646	92950
36000-36015	92953
36120-36140	92960
35400-35440	93000-93018
36600-36619	93307-93325†
36621-36624	93922-93981†
36626-36640	94640
62278-62279†	94650
64400-64565	94651
67500	94656†
80002-80202	94660-94662†
81000-81050	94664-94665
82000-87253	94680-94690
88104-88182	94760-94770
89050-89365	99201-99499
90780-90788	

The daggered codes on this list must not be confused with "starred" procedures in CPT. The daggered codes can be billed separately in the following situations:

- **Epidural block codes 62274-66279.** These codes may be billed on the date of surgery if performed for postoperative pain relief and not used as anesthesia during a surgical procedure. When this service is provided on the day of surgery, a modifier is used to indicate a distinct procedure and a separate procedure note is included in the medical record.
- **Echocardiography codes 93307-93325.** These codes may be reported in addition to anesthesia time when performed for diagnostic purposes (not monitoring) with documentation including a formal report.
- **Extremity arterial venous study codes 93922-93981.** These codes may be reported if they are for diagnostic purposes and a formal report has been prepared.
- **Ventilation management and pulmonary services code 94656 and codes 94660-94662.** These codes may be separately reported if performed after transfer out of the postanesthesia unit to ICU. Modifier-59 should be appended to the CPT code to show that it is a distinct service. When ventilation management is provided during surgery, it is included in the anesthesia service.

SURGERY GUIDELINES

Basic guidelines for reporting of surgical procedure codes in CPT are found in the CPT manual. Reporting requirements for reimbursement are dependent on the carrier involved. Many surgical procedures are reported and billed according to a global fee concept. This "package" of services may not be the same as a CPT-defined surgical package. According to the Surgery Guidelines that precede the Surgery section of the manual, "Listed surgical procedures include the operation per se, local infiltration, metacarpal/digital block, or topical anesthesia when used, and normal uncomplicated follow-up care." Follow-up services that are part of a global package should be reported using code 99024 (postoperative follow-up visit, included in global service). No charge is associated with this code, since the global fee includes this part of the service.

Using the CPT definition, it would always be incorrect to unbundle routine postoperative services and administration of local anesthesia as a service for additional payment from an insurance plan.

Using the CPT definition, it would always be incorrect to unbundle routine postoperative services and administration of local anesthesia as a service for additional payment from an insurance plan. Many health insurance plans also will not allow separate payment for an office "visit" at the same time as a procedure code, unless significant separately identifiable services are provided that are not a part of the global concept.

HCFA and possibly some other carriers define global periods as 0 days, 10 days (minor procedures), or 90 days (major procedures). Medicare's billing policy requires that a single fee be billed and reimbursement provided for all necessary services normally furnished by the surgeon before, during, and after the procedure. Major surgery usually has a collection of services that occur on separate days but are all part of the same global fee. For global billing the services rendered are reported on a claim with the date of surgery or maternal delivery listed as the date of service. There are selected items that may be reported separately. When these occur they should be reported on a separate claim with the appropriate dates.

Postoperative follow-up visit, included in global service

Global Surgery Concepts for Third Party Reimbursement

Included in Medicare global fees are:

- Visits to the patient after the decision to operate has been made, beginning with the day before surgery for major procedures and the day of surgery for minor procedures. This would mean that extra visits to educate or prepare the patient for surgery would not be billed over and above the surgery fee.
- Services that occur intraoperatively and are normally part of the surgery itself.
- Services for complications that do not require an additional trip to the operating room. This may not be the rule for other types of insurance plans that use the CPT definition that states "normal uncomplicated care" is included in the global concept. Some plans allow for reimbursement of services to take care of complications, particularly for maternity services that are not routine.
- 90 days of care after the surgery if the care is related to the diagnosis that prompted the operation. Minor surgeries are only 10 days or may have 0 follow-up days. Other health plans may have different follow-up periods in a global fee structure for surgical services.

The following list is for HCFA services that are not included in the global fee. In general, reporting of these services separately should be appropriate for most other health plans.

- The initial consultation or evaluation of the problem by the surgeon where the physician discusses with the patient the need for surgery. Medicare pays for this even if no surgery occurs. Modifier -57 may be appended if the date of this decision is the day before or the day of surgery.
- History/physical exam performed more than a day before the surgery date. Separate reimbursement is paid to a family practice physician or internist to "clear" the patient for surgery or to perform the admitting H&P required for hospital admission. When the surgeon performs this service it is not separately paid.
- Reoperations for complications requiring a return trip to the operating room. Medicare doesn't duplicate the reimbursement for preoperative and postoperative services but will pay for the operative portion (the operation per se). If no CPT code existed for the reoperation, it couldn't be billed for more the 50 percent of the initial surgery charge according to Medicare rules.
- Added treatments that are not part of normal recovery from surgery.
- Immunosuppressive drug therapy for organ transplants.
- Dialysis, both inpatient and outpatient.
- Critical care services (codes 99291, 99292) which are unrelated to the surgery and require constant attendance of the physician.
- Treatment for postoperative complications which require a return trip to the operating room. If the physician reporting is not the ER physician who initially performed the work, separate payment can be obtained without reducing the ER physician's allowed amount.
- Selected services allow reporting of a surgical tray in addition to the code for the procedure. Splints and casting supplies may be reported separately from other services. These are reimbursed under the "reasonable charge" payment system.
- Services of other physicians except when the services included in a global package are furnished by more than one physician (i.e., group practice visits that share hospital calls following surgery).
- Diagnostic tests and procedures, including diagnostic radiology procedures.
- Clearly distinct surgical procedures during the postoperative period which aren't reoperations or treatment for complications. A new postoperative period begins with any subsequent procedure.

- Visit services (E/M codes) unrelated to the diagnosis for which the surgical procedure is performed. Modifier -24 may be added to assure the service is not denied, despite the different diagnosis codes. A distinct ICD-9-CM code is often the key to separate reimbursement for these services.

Follow-Up Care for Diagnostic Procedures

The CPT code assigned for diagnostic procedures such as endoscopy, arthroscopy, injection procedures for radiology, etc., includes only the care related to the diagnostic procedure itself. Care of the condition that required the performance of the procedure is not included in this service and should be reported separately for appropriate reimbursement.

EXAMPLE

If a patient with reflux esophagitis is examined with an endoscope in the hospital outpatient department on Monday to confirm the diagnosis and rule out esophageal ulcers and returns to the physician's office on Wednesday due to hematemesis, the office service may be reported separately because it is not related to performance of the endoscopy.

Follow-Up Care for Therapeutic Surgical Procedures

CPT guidelines include only the care that is routinely part of the surgical service. Additional services required for complications, exacerbation, etc., should be separately reported as they occur. Medicare has specific limitations on paying for follow-up care, even for complications, when they are surgery-related. Other insurance plans may have varying rules for payment of complications related to surgery.

Supplies and Materials

CPT allows separate reporting for supplies or materials that are usually included in an office visit. Examples include drugs, surgical trays, special bandages, and durable medical equipment stocked in the office. CPT has only one code for supplies (99070). Many third party payers will not reimburse for services reported with this code without a detailed description. HCPCS codes allow more concise reporting of these items. Many health plans consider routine supplies included in office visit codes or minor procedure codes and will not provide separate payment. Such things must be considered when establishing a fee or a cost allocation study for services listed by CPT codes. Hospitals often assign CPT and/or HCPCS codes to supplies and materials for data management and charging purposes. In the APC system, supplies and materials will most often be "packaged" into the APC group and not separately reimbursed by Medicare or other payers using the APC system.

Multiple Procedures

It is always appropriate to designate multiple procedures that are rendered on the same day by using separate entries and CPT codes. For reimbursement purposes, however, the codes may be bundled together or the value reduced to eliminate duplication of the allowance for preoperative and postoperative services. Modifier -51 is often used on subsequent procedures for physician billing. Use of this modifier is described in detail in Chapter 8.

Add-On Codes

There are quite a few codes in the CPT system that are commonly carried out in addition to the primary procedure reported. All add-on codes found in CPT are exempt from the multiple procedure concept and should not be modified. These codes often include the words "each additional" or similar language and would never stand alone, since the primary procedure would always be reported first. Often the phrase "List separately in addition to primary procedure" is found after the code description. In 1999, the add-on codes are marked with the + symbol.

Separate Procedure Designation

Some of the procedures in CPT are commonly carried out as an integral part of a total service or procedure and have been identified by the addition of the words "separate procedure" in the description. Codes with this designation should not be reported in addition to codes for the total procedure or service that they may be part of. When one of these procedures is performed independent of, or distinct from, other procedures, it may be appropriate to report it separately. Modifier -59 is sometimes used for reporting a separate procedure code in this situation to prevent third party payer denials as a bundled service. Additional information is available in Chapter 8 about the use of modifier -59. In normal circumstances a "separate procedure" code will be reported without other procedure codes on the claim.

"Unlisted Procedure" Codes

CPT provides a way to report procedures that do not have a specific code by having "unlisted procedure" codes available in each section. A listing of the current unlisted procedure codes is found within the section guidelines in the CPT manual. When a service or procedure is performed and no code is available, the provider selects the unlisted procedure code from the CPT section that, if a code existed, would be found in that section. For example, a keyhole coronary artery bypass procedure performed via laparoscope does not have its own CPT code. Therefore the unlisted procedure code from the laparoscopy section is assigned (56399). Because unlisted procedure codes vary widely from case to case, any third party payer will want documentation of what was done in detail so that it can be priced appropriately for reimbursement. A letter from the physician stating the difficulty, risk, and equipment required for the procedure is recommended along with a copy of the actual operative report so that the best possible payment for the work performed is granted. If information is not available for optimal pricing, payment from the insurance company will not be what is expected or deserved.

Starred Procedures

An asterisk "✻" or star next to a CPT code indicates that according to CPT conventions, the "surgical package" concept does not apply to these codes due to wide variance in preoperative and postoperative service needs. Therefore the code denotes only the operative portion of the procedure and the reporting provider is free to add on preoperative and postoperative visits as necessary. According to the manual, when a star follows the surgical procedure code the following rules apply:

1. The service as listed includes only the surgical procedures. Associated pre- and postoperative services are not included in the service as listed.

2. Preoperative services are considered as one of the following:

**Initial (new patient)
visit when starred
(✳) procedure
constitutes major
service at that visit**

When the starred procedure is carried out at the time of an initial visit (new patient) and this procedure constitutes the major service at that visit, procedure code 99025 is listed in lieu of the usual initial visit as an additional service.

When the starred procedure is carried out at the time of an initial or other visit involving significant identifiable services (e.g., removal of a small skin lesion at the time of a comprehensive history and physical examination), the appropriate visit is listed in addition to the starred procedures and its follow-up care.

When the starred procedure is carried out at the time of a follow-up (established patient) visit and this procedure constitutes the major service at that visit, the service visit is usually not added.

When the starred procedure requires hospitalization, an appropriate hospital visit is listed in addition to the starred procedure and its follow-up care.

3. All postoperative care is added on a service-by-service basis (e.g., hospital visit, cast change).
4. Complications are added on a service-by-service basis (as with all surgical procedures).

Although these rules are true for CPT, Medicare and some other payers do not recognize or reimburse according to the starred procedure rules. For Medicare reporting, surgery codes are priced to include preoperative and postoperative services. When services over and above the normal activities surrounding a minor procedure occur and the documentation supports the claim that the services were significant and separately identifiable, separate reimbursement may be obtained by use of modifier -25 on the E/M code. Code 99025 is not a payable code for Medicare reimbursement.

Surgical Destruction

Surgical destruction is a part of a surgical procedure and different methods of destruction are not ordinarily listed separately unless the technique employed substantially alters the usual management of a problem or condition. When there are exceptions for special circumstances, separate code numbers are provided.

INTEGUMENTARY SYSTEM

The CPT codes in the Integumentary System section (10040-19499) are used by a number of physician specialties. The coding system is oriented towards dermatology including closure, tissue transfer, skin grafts, and adjacent and distant flap grafts. Procedures in the Integumentary System contain a number of "add-on" codes and are often performed in stages due to the sophistication of the surgical techniques used.

Evaluation and Management of integumentary disorders may represent a separately identifiable service since it may serve as an encounter where a decision is made for a surgical procedure and is significant enough and distinct enough to warrant separate reporting. Generally, if the E/M service is for the decision to perform surgery, it is established as a significant, separately identifiable service and may be reported in addition to the surgical code for a single encounter. Reimbursement rules vary by health plan and documentation should always support the separate service over and above normal preoperative activities.

Surgical dressings, supplies, and local anesthesia used for integumentary procedures are often not separately reportable, as health plans consider these services to be bundled with the procedure.

Incision and Drainage

Incision and drainage (I&D) services usually involve cutaneous or subcutaneous drainage of cysts, pustules, infections, hematomas, seromas, or fluid collections. In the case where excision of a lesion is performed in conjunction with I&D, or the I&D is performed to gain access to the area of the lesion, it would be inappropriate to code both procedures. Only the code for the excision should be reported.

> ### EXAMPLE
>
> A patient with a pilonidal cyst may require a simple incision and drainage or in more extensive cases, an excision of the cyst. For a simple I&D, code 10080✱ is reported. Since this is a "starred" procedure in CPT, appropriate preoperative and postoperative services may be added. If the pilonidal cyst is more problematic, excision may be required. It is obvious that incision and drainage will be accomplished during the excision of the cyst, but the code assignment will be 11770, 11771, or 11772 depending on the nature of the service.

Procedure codes such as I&D of hematomas (10140✱) are not reported separately when performed with excision, repair, destruction, removal, etc., since the latter procedures are more comprehensive and include the incision and drainage integral to the other work.

Lesion Removal

When coding lesion removal in CPT, the size and the nature of the lesion must be known. It is important not to assign codes without the operative report and pathology report available for this reason. When possible, the size of the lesion should be obtained from the operative report rather than the pathology description, since shrinkage or fragmentation of tissue may occur. The size of the defect is never reported for CPT coding purposes, only the actual size of the lesion. Because CPT codes are classified in centimeters, this is the unit of measure that must be used in code selection. The size of lesion is measured by its diameter in a circular or ellipse lesion (see Figure 7.1). The diameter is the length of a straight line segment passing through the center of a figure (circle or sphere) and terminating at the perimeter. Lesions may not be "added up" like repair codes. Each lesion requiring attention is separately reportable unless the code includes multiple lesion removal in a single procedure code.

FIGURE 7.1   Lesion Measurement: Excision Malignant Lesion of Face .6 cm, Code 11641

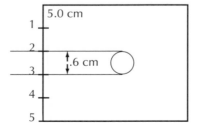

For a given lesion, only one type of removal is reported, whether it is destruction by laser or freezing, debridement, paring, curettement, shaving, or excision by scalpel. In the event of an initial attempt made with a less invasive procedure that is converted to a more invasive procedure, the more complex procedure is coded, not both procedures. Multiple codes describing destruction of a lesion are not to be assigned for a given lesion. If there are multiple methods used for multiple lesions of differing natures,

> *For a given lesion, only one type of removal is reported, whether it is destruction by laser or freezing, debridement, paring, curettement, shaving, or excision by scalpel.*

then a modifier such as -59 is used to explain the use of multiple codes.

A lesion biopsy represents a partial removal of a lesion and may be performed as part of a lesion excision to obtain a pathological specimen for diagnosis. When a biopsy is performed as part of a lesion removal, the biopsy should be considered incident to the excision and not reported separately. When the biopsy is performed at a separate operative session and then subsequently the lesion is removed, perhaps on a different date, separate reporting is appropriate.

Surgical Pathology codes

Qualified physicians in dermatopathology may perform surgical pathological evaluation in addition to lesion biopsy or excision. To report these services, CPT codes 88300-83309 from the Surgical Pathology section are used.

Lesion removal by various methods, generally excisional, often requires simple, intermediate, or complex closure or in some circumstances tissue transfer procedures. When the lesion removal requires strip closure or simple sutures involving only the skin, this is included in the lesion removal and is not reported separately. Intermediate and complex closures require separate reporting using the appropriate CPT codes for layer closure. See the section on repair for additional coding tips.

Intralesional Chemotherapy

Injection of neoplastic agents Other intralesional therapy

CPT codes 96405 and 96406 are used to report injection of anti-neoplastic agents into one or multiple lesions. CPT codes 11900 and 11901 are used for other types of intralesional therapy not described as chemotherapy. Code 11900 may be used for injecting one to seven lesions. The code is reported only once even if a particular lesion is injected more than once. The 96405-96406 codes would not normally be reported with the 11900-11901 codes. In the case of separate lesions injected with different agents, modifier -59 would be used to report the separate service. These CPT codes are included in the following list of other services and would not be reported in addition:

1. 11200-11201   Removal of Skin Tags
2. 11300-11313   Shaving of Lesions
3. 11400-11471   Excision of Benign Lesions
4. 11600-11646   Excision of Malignant Lesions
5. 11765   Wedge Excision
6. 11719-11772   Excision, Debridement, and Excision of Nails, Pilonidal Cysts
7. 12001-12018   Simple Repairs
8. 12020-12021   Treatment of Wound Dehiscence
9. 12031-12057   Intermediate Repairs
10. 13100-13300   Complex Repairs

Adjacent tissue transfer and/or tissue rearrangement

When a lesion excision is so extensive that closure cannot be obtained by normal suturing, other techniques may be employed, including adjacent tissue transfer and/or tissue rearrangement. This section of codes from 14000-14350 involves excision with adjacent tissue transfer and correlates to excision codes. The lesion removal and repairs are not coded separately in these procedures, nor is debridement. Skin grafting codes may be separately reported only when the skin graft is not included in the specific procedure code description under consideration.

Repairs

Repair of skin wounds may be classified as simple, intermediate, or complex. CPT guidelines preceding codes 12001-13300 state:

Simple repair is used when the wound is superficial; e.g., involving primarily epidermis or dermis, or subcutaneous tissues without significant involvement of deeper tissues and requires simple one layer closure/suturing. Local anesthesia and electrocauterization of wounds is included in simple closure. Closure with adhesive strips is not coded as simple closure, but is included in the appropriate Evaluation and Management service of the physician.

Simple repair

Intermediate repair includes the repair of wounds that require layered closure of one or more of the deeper layers of subcutaneous tissue and superficial (non-muscle) fascia, in addition to the skin (epidermal and dermal) closure. Single layer closure of heavily contaminated wounds that have required extensive cleaning or removal of particulate matter also constitutes intermediate repair.

Intermediate repair

Complex repair includes the repair of wounds requiring more than layered closure such as scar revision, debridement of traumatic lacerations or avulsion, extensive undermining, stents, or retention sutures. It may include creation of the defect and necessary preparation for repairs or the debridement and repair of complicated lacerations.

Complex repair

Instructions for reporting services at the time of wound repair:

1. The repaired wound should be measured and recorded in centimeters, whether curved, angular, or stellate.
2. When multiple wounds are repaired, add together those in the same classification and report as a single item. When more than one classification of wounds is repaired, list the more complicated as the primary procedure and the less complicated as the secondary procedure, using modifier -51 (00951) on the second procedure.
3. Decontamination and/or debridement is considered a separate procedure only when gross contamination requires prolonged cleansing, when appreciable amounts of devitalized or contaminated tissue are removed, or when debridement is carried out separately without immediate primary closure. For extensive debridement of soft tissue and/or bone, CPT codes 11040-11044 may be reported as appropriate. When extensive debridement of subcutaneous tissue, muscle fascia, muscle, and/or bone associated with open fracture(s) and/or dislocation(s) are performed, codes 11010-11012 should be considered.

   Extensive debridement of soft tissue and/or bone

4. Involvement of nerves, blood vessels, and tendons are reported under the appropriate system (Nervous, Cardiovascular, Musculoskeletal) rather than coded as wound repairs. The wound repair for these procedures is included in the primary procedure code unless it qualifies as a complex wound, in which case modifier -51 would be added to the wound repair code for multiple procedure designation.
5. Simple ligation of vessels in an open wound is considered part of wound closure and should not be separately reported.
6. Simple "exploration" of nerves, blood vessels, or tendons exposed in an open wound is also considered part of the essential treatment of the wound and is not a separate procedure unless appreciable dissection is required. If the wound requires any of the following, use codes 20100-20103, as appropriate.

Exploration of penetrating wounds

- Enlargement, extension of the dissection (to determine penetration)
- Debridement, removal of foreign body(s)
- Ligation or coagulation of minor subcutaneous and/or muscular blood vessels of the subcutaneous tissues, muscle fascia, and/or muscle, not requiring thoracotomy or laparotomy

Debridement

In the course of destruction, excision, incision, removal, and repair of the skin, debridement of the nonviable tissue surrounding the lesion or injury is often necessary in conjunction with the primary service. These codes (11000-11042) are not separately reported unless the debridement is extensive and requires prolonged work separate from the other procedure. Modifier -59 should be used when reporting debridement with a primary procedure and the documentation within the medical record must support the separately identifiable service.

Skin Grafts

CPT includes codes for Adjacent Tissue Transfer and Rearrangement, Free Skin Grafts, Skin Flaps, and Other Flaps and Grafts. Coding tips for each section follow. There is a "ladder of reconstruction" that helps to picture how wounds are cared for depending on the type, location of the defect on the body, and what tissue is available for use.

Adjacent Tissue Transfer 14000-14350

When a lesion is excised and tissue from an adjacent site is transferred, the excision of the lesion is not coded separately since it is included in the transfer code. The size of the tissue should be obtained in square centimeters. Debridement to accomplish tissue transfers is also included in the code. Lacerations that coincidentally are approximated using a tissue transfer technique such as Z-plasty or W-plasty should be reported using the closure code. **Eyelid procedures** Eyelid procedures have their own codes for reconstruction using tissue transfers such as 67961-67966.

Free Skin Grafts 15000-15400

Free skin grafts Free skin grafts include punch graphs, split thickness grafts, full-thickness grafts, allografts, and zenografts. Preparation of the recipient site and repair of the donor site should be determined before code assignment. Repair of the donor site is reported as an additional procedure. When more extensive procedures are performed such as orbitectomy or radical mastectomy, the primary procedure is coded first, followed by a code from this section for the skin grafting.

Free skin grafts are coded by type (split or full), location, and size. For each location, a primary code is defined and followed by a supplemental code for any additional coverage area required. For reporting on the HCFA 1500, the initial code would be limited to one unit of service but the supplemental code may have multiple units depending on the extent of the area.

In general, debridement of non-intact skin in anticipation of a graft is included in the **Preparation of** code. When skin is intact and the graft is performed following excisional preparation of **recipient site** intact skin, the excisional preparation code (15000) is reported separately. This code is not intended to describe debridement of necrotic or infected skin, nor is its use indicated with other lesion removal codes.

CPT code 15350 for application of allograft and 15400 for application of xenograft are part of all other graft codes and would not be separately reported with other grafts in the range of 15050-15261 for graft placement on the same location.

Allograft
Xenograft

Flap Grafts 15570-15776

The type of flap and recipient location must be determined before coding. If a microvascular anastomosis was performed, codes 15756-15758 should be referenced. If the donor site required skin graft or repair, an additional code should be reported. When extensive mobilization is documented, the appropriate other sections of CPT should be consulted. Large plaster casts and other immobilizing devices are considered separate procedures and are reported in addition to the flap codes.

Microvascular anastomosis

Microvascular Transfers

When tissues are transferred from one body site to another using microsurgery techniques, these are coded differently than flap grafts. The term "free" is used to indicate that the tissue is separated from its blood supply and transferred to a recipient site where it is reconnected to the recipient blood vessels. Other flaps remain attached to their blood supply. The free tissue transfer codes include transferring a portion of the fascia which contains the vascular supply to the skin.

Code 15756 is used to report free muscle flaps with or without skin with microvascular anastomosis. Coverage of a free muscle flap is not always accomplished at the same time as the free flap, and therefore should be coded separately. In a case where there is a free muscle flap combined with its overlying skin, there would be no skin graft applied to the muscle and no additional code would be necessary. If the muscle is applied without the skin, then a skin graft would be later applied and would require separate coding. The preparation and debridement of the recipient site prior to the actual creation and transfer flap (which include the microdissection of arteries, veins, and nerves) are not included in the free flap graft code and can be reported separately. Separate codes may also be assigned in the case where skin graft is needed to close the donor muscle flap site. The donor site will always be closed at the time of the free flap, either directly or with a skin graft, and this will be reported separately by using codes 15000-15400.

Free muscle flaps

Breast Procedures

Because of the unique nature of procedures developed to address breast disease, a section of CPT in the Integumentary section is set aside for reporting these procedures. Codes 19000-19499 are used for reporting breast procedures.

Fine needle aspiration biopsies, core biopsies, open biopsies, and related procedures performed to procure tissue from a lesion for which an established diagnosis exists are not reported separately at the time of lesion excision unless the biopsy is performed on a different lesion or on the other breast. If a diagnosis is not established at the time of the biopsy and the decision to perform the surgery is dependent on the results, then it is appropriate to assign both codes.

Breast procedures

Because excision of lesions are inherent in the course of a mastectomy, they are not separately coded. CPT codes 19101-19126 are included within the mastectomy codes. Codes for incision and closure are included in the codes describing the various breast excision or mastectomy procedures. A biopsy of lymph nodes or muscle tissue excision in conjunction with mastectomy is included in the mastectomy codes. CPT codes for breast procedures refer primarily to unilateral procedures. When performed on both breasts at one session, the bilateral modifier -50 would be appropriate.

Excision of breast lesions

MUSCULOSKELETAL SYSTEM

This section of CPT includes wound exploration for trauma, excision of musculoskeletal structures, introduction and removal of materials from bones, joints, and muscles, replantation procedures, graft procedures, fracture care, and a variety of repair procedures and reconstruction surgery.

Procedure codes in the Musculoskeletal System section include the application and removal of the first cast or traction device only. If a cast and/or traction device must be subsequently replaced, then an additional code may be assigned.

Fracture Care Reporting

Application of casts and strapping

Fracture therapy generally falls into a global surgery concept for reimbursement to physicians. Therefore, preoperative, operative, and normal postoperative care is represented by the CPT code for fracture care. There may be times when a physician provides initial stabilization of a fracture before restorative treatment is completed by an orthopedic physician. The Application of Casts and Strapping guidelines found in the CPT book instruct coders to use the code range 29000-29799 for the following:

- a replacement cast/strapping procedure, during or after the period of normal follow-up care
- an initial service performed without restorative treatment or procedures to stabilize or protect a fracture, injury or dislocation, and/or to afford pain relief to a patient
- an initial cast/strapping service when no other treatment or procedure is performed or expected to be performed by the same physician
- an initial cast/strapping service, when another physician provides a restorative treatment or procedure

Therefore, it is appropriate for an emergency department physician to assign a CPT code for application of cast or strapping in addition to the E/M code (assuming the key components are met for E/M service). Hospitals would assign a fracture therapy code if fracture reduction were accomplished in the emergency department by the ED physician or through an outpatient surgical procedure by another physician.

Fractures are treated by closed reduction techniques, open treatment methods, and percutaneous skeletal fixation. Closed treatment means that the fracture site is not surgically exposed to the external environment and directly visualized. CPT defines closed treatments for these three methods:

1. without manipulation
2. with manipulation
3. with or without traction

Manipulation is used throughout the musculoskeletal fracture and dislocation subsections of CPT to specifically mean the attempted reduction or restoration of a fracture or joint dislocation to its normal anatomic alignment by application of manually applied forces.

Open treatment is used for surgical repair when the fracture is exposed to the external environment. The bone break is visualized and internal fixation may be used to reduce the fracture.

In general, the application of external immobilization devices (including casts) after a procedure includes the maintenance and removal services during the global fee period.

Additional CPT codes are provided for removal and modification of external fixation devices by physicians other than the physician who applied the device and for hospital use.

Supplies used in casting are separately reported using CPT supply code 99070 or the appropriate HCPCS code. CPT codes describing modification of casts (29700-29750) would not be reported when modifications are performed at the same time as the initial fracture care services.

CPT supply code

Percutaneous skeletal fixation is a technique that is neither open nor closed fracture treatment. For this type of fracture care the fracture fragments are not visualized, but a fixation device such as a pin(s) is placed across the fracture, usually with the assistance of X-ray imaging guidance.

The type of fracture coded in ICD-9-CM does not have any direct coding correlation with the type of treatment used, but may correspond in some circumstances. For example, an open fracture is usually repaired by an open reduction, but a closed fracture may be treated with open reduction and internal fixation as well.

Reimbursement policies often have rules about "most extensive" procedures that state that when a fracture requires closed reduction followed by open reduction during the same patient encounter, only the open reduction service is eligible for reimbursement.

Skeletal traction is defined as a force (distracting or traction force) to a limb segment through a wire, pin, screw, or clamp that is attached to (e.g., penetrates) the bone. Separate codes have been created for removal of internal fixation devices as a separate procedure and modification/removal of these devices in conjunction with another procedure. When a superficial or deep implant requires surgery for removal, it may be reported as a separate procedure. If this service is performed in conjunction with another procedure involving the same area it would not be appropriate to report it separately for reimbursement.

Skin traction is the application of a force to a limb using felt or strapping applied to skin only without bone involvement.

External fixation employs the use of skeletal pins plus an attaching mechanism/device for either temporary or definitive treatment of acute or chronic bone deformity.

CPT codes for obtaining autogenous bone grafts, cartilage, tendons, fascia lata grafts, or other tissues through separate incisions are to be used only when the graft is not already listed as part of the basic procedure. Also the codes for external fixation are to be used only when external fixation is not listed as part of the basic procedure.

For facial fractures where interdental wiring (e.g., CPT code 21497) is required, third party payers may mandate inclusion for this work as part of the primary service (reconstructive surgery or arthroplasty). When reported with other head and neck procedures, modifier -59 may be used to denote a distinctly separate procedure. Medical record documentation in this case should substantiate the separately identifiable service.

Interdental wiring

Codes with 10 days or 0 follow-up days in the global period will require a modifier (i.e., -25) for separate reporting of an ER visit and fracture care by the same physician.

Hospitals may assign fracture care codes even when no fracture reduction procedure is performed if the fracture therapy care is well documented. However, many hospitals have a coding protocol where if no manipulation, bone setting, or service is used, then only the emergency room or outpatient department visit code is reported.

Electrical Stimulation for Bone Healing

Codes 20974-20975 should be assigned for electrical stimulation for bone healing. The codes for nerve stimulation are not used for this purpose. If a neurostimulator is medically necessary for pain control or other conditions, modifier -59 should be used to show that the service is separate and represents treatment for different symptoms. CPT codes 97014 and 97032 from the Physical Medicine section should not be reported with codes in this range.

Electrical stimulation for bone healing

Physical therapy modalities

Debridement

Debridement of fracture codes should only be assigned in addition to fracture therapy codes when the debridement is extensive or is directed at concurrent tissue damage due to trauma. While these debridement codes are intended to be used in cases of open fractures, there may be examples when debridement is necessary to treat a fracture site when no open fracture is present. In a traumatic fracture the skin could be damaged extensively and involve surrounding tissues. Significant debridement could be required even though the wound is not involved down to the fracture and then it would be appropriate to utilize the appropriate code from the 11010-11012 range.

Debridement of open fractures

Graft Codes

Bone, cartilage, tendon, and other types of grafts are only separately coded if the major procedure does not include the graft within its definition. Spinal procedures require separate reporting of autografts obtained. These procedures are add-on procedures and would not be reported as multiple procedures using modifier -51. If bone marrow is aspirated for grafting, code 85095 is separately listed to report the aspiration. The placement of the bone marrow aspirate is included in the arthrodesis procedure and would not be coded in addition to the other procedures.

Bone marrow aspiration

Instrumentation for Spinal Procedures

Arthrodesis and spinal surgery

Codes 22840-22848 and 22851 should be reported separately in addition to codes for the fracture, dislocation, or arthrodesis of the spine (CPT codes 22324, 22326, 22327, and 22548-22812). It is important to note that code 22851 is not intended to be reported per cage. Only if cages are placed at two different levels (e.g., at L3-4 interspace and L5-S1 interspace) should the code be used more than once. A single cage may replace three entire vertebrae, wherein code 22851 would be only reported once.

When arthrodesis is performed in addition to another procedure, the arthrodesis should be reported in addition to the original procedure with the modifier -51 appended for multiple procedures. Examples include arthrodesis after osteotomy, fracture care, vertebral corpectomy, and laminectomy. Because bone grafts and instrumentation are never performed without arthrodesis, they are reported as add-on codes and modifier -51 is not used. More information about modifier use is found in Chapter 8.

RESPIRATORY SYSTEM

Respiratory system procedures

Respiratory System procedures are reported using codes in the 30000-39999 range. Because the upper airway is bordered by mucocutaneous margins, there are several CPT codes to report services involving biopsy, destruction, excision, and removal procedures for lesions of this margin in the nasal and oral surfaces. When reporting these services, the CPT code which describes the services performed should be reported from either the Integumentary System or the Respiratory System sections. When the narrative description accompanying the CPT codes from the Respiratory Section includes tissue transfer such as grafts, flaps, etc., it would not be appropriate to also assign codes from the 14000-15770 range.

When a biopsy is obtained as part of the excision, destruction, or other types of removal either by endoscopy or by incision at the same session, a biopsy code would not be separately reported. In the case where the decision to perform a more comprehensive surgery is dependent on the results of the biopsy, it would be appropriate to separately list the biopsy code.

EXAMPLE

In a patient with nasal obstruction, sinus obstruction, and nasal polyps, a biopsy may be required prior to or in conjunction with a polypectomy and ethmoidectomy. A separate code such as 31237 (nasal endoscopy) would not be reported with the more comprehensive endoscopy code 31255 even though the comprehensive code does not specifically list a biopsy in the CPT narrative.

When a diagnostic endoscopy is performed, it is included in any of the more comprehensive surgical endoscopy codes and is not separately reported. For example, fiberoptic bronchoscopy services will routinely include inspection of the nasal cavity, the pharynx, and the larynx. Only the code for the bronchoscopy would be assigned, and no additional codes for the nasal endoscopy or laryngoscopy would be reported unless separately carried out. Some third party payers allow reporting of a diagnostic endoscopy in addition to the surgical procedure when the diagnostic endoscopy results in a decision to perform the surgery. Modifier -59 is used to show that the surgical procedure service is distinct from the diagnostic procedure.

Sinus Procedures

When a sinusotomy is performed in conjunction with a sinus endoscopy, only one service is assigned a CPT code. Surgical sinus endoscopy always includes a sinusotomy and a diagnostic endoscopy by CPT definition. Multiple endoscopic procedures may be separately reported when no single comprehensive code adequately describes what was done, such as may occur with FESS (Functional Endoscopic Sinus Surgery). Incidental examination of other areas by endoscope in addition to the primary procedure does not warrant separate coding and reporting.

Sinus surgeries may involve one or more of the four sinus cavities on each side. Since these sinuses are separate anatomic locations and there is separate identifiable work in each sinus, all areas must be coded for optimal reimbursement. CPT codes 31231-31294 are used to report unilateral procedures unless otherwise specified in the documentation. If one of the procedures listed in this range is performed bilaterally, and the code description does not specify bilateral procedure, then modifier -50 may be appended to the code. Codes reported in addition to the primary procedure should have modifier -51 appended. Please refer to Chapter 8 for detailed information about CPT Modifiers.

Sinus surgeries

Other Respiratory Procedures

When *laryngoscopy* is required for placement of an endotracheal tube, the laryngoscopy code is omitted from reporting. Code 31500 refers only to endotracheal intubation as an emergency procedure which is not reported when electively performed in conjunction with general anesthesia or bronchoscopy. When intubation is performed for a rapidly deteriorating patient requiring mechanical ventilation assistance, a separate code is appropriate for the intubation.

Laryngoscopy

When a *tracheostomy* is performed as an essential part of laryngeal surgery, CPT code 31600 would not be separately reported since it is included in the more comprehensive procedures. Also, when the laryngoscopy is required for the placement of a tracheostomy, the tracheostomy (CPT codes 31603-31614) would be reported, not the laryngoscopy.

Tracheostomy

Code 92511 (nasopharyngoscopy with endoscopy) from the Medicine section of CPT is included in the respiratory endoscopy procedures when performed at the same session and would not be separately reported.

Nasopharyngoscopy with endoscopy

Thoracentesis   *Thoracentesis* is reported using a CPT code in the range of 32000-32020. Insertion of chest tubes for drainage purposes is coded in this section when reported separately from more comprehensive thoracic surgery. A tube thoracostomy (insertion of chest tube) is assigned to code 32020.

CARDIOVASCULAR SYSTEM

CPT coding in the cardiovascular system requires detailed knowledge of cardiac and vascular system anatomy and physiology and attention to specific coding guidelines. Selective vascular catheterization should be coded to include introduction of the catheter and all lesser order selective catheterizations used in the approach. For example, the code description for a selective right middle cerebral artery catheterization includes the introduction and placement catheterization of the right common and internal carotid arteries. Additional second and/or third order arterial catheterizations within the same family of arteries supplied by a single first order artery should be expressed by assignment of code 36218 or 36248.

Arterial catheterizations   Additional first order or higher catheterizations in vascular families supplied by first order vessels different from a previously selected and coded family should be separately coded using the conventions described above, according to the CPT manual.

Pacemakers and Defibrillators

For pacemaker or defibrillator placement, it must be known whether the procedure is an initial service or a replacement and the specific type of the device must be documented for accurate code assignment. A pacemaker always includes a pulse generator and one or more electrode "leads" inserted in one of several ways. Pulse generators may be placed in a subcutaneous fashioned "pocket" created in a subclavicular or intra-abdominal location. Electrodes may be inserted through a vein (transvenous) or on the surface of the heart (epicardial). When a single chamber system is used, a pulse generator and one electrode are inserted in either the atrium or the ventricle of the heart. A dual chamber system also has a pulse generator, but one electrode is inserted in the atrium and one electrode is inserted in the ventricle.

Defibrillator systems also include a pulse generator and electrodes for implantation. The pulse generator may be placed in a subcutaneous pocket and the electrodes will be inserted either transvenously or epicardially.

When the medical record documents a battery change, it is the pulse generator that is being replaced. Replacement of the pulse generator for pacemaker or defibrillator systems requires assignment of a code for removal of the pulse generator and another code for the insertion of the new one. Repositioning within the first 14 days of the insertion or replacement is included in the service and would not be reported again per the CPT manual instructions.

CABG Procedure Coding

Coronary artery bypass grafts   When a coronary artery bypass is performed, the most comprehensive code describing the procedure is the one that should be reported. Only one code in the range of codes 33510-33516 (venous grafting) and no other bypass codes are correctly reported with these codes. One code in the range of code 33517-33523 (combined arterial-venous grafting) and one in the range of 33533-33536 (arterial grafting) can be billed together to accurately describe combined arterial-venous bypass. When only arterial grafting is performed, one code from the range of 33533-33536 is reported.

When a median sternotomy is performed to accomplish cardiothoracic procedures, the repair of the sternal incision is part of the primary procedure. CPT codes 21820-21825 (treatment of sternum fracture) are not reported separately, nor would it be appropriate for a physician to separately code removal of embedded wires should a repeat procedure be performed.

Procurement of a venous graft is integral to the performance of coronary artery bypass employing venous grafts and is not reported separately with a CPT code. Therefore CPT codes in the range of 37700-37775 (ligation of saphenous veins) would not be assigned when codes 33510-33523 are reported for the primary procedure.

When an intervascular shunt procedure is performed as a part of another procedure requiring vascular revision, the service for the shunt procedure is not separately coded from CPT code range 36800-36861 (intervascular cannulization/shunt). CPT has designated these procedures as "separate procedures."

Aneurysm repair may require direct repair with or without graft insertion or use thromboendarterectomy and/or bypass techniques. When a thromboendarterectomy is undertaken at the site of the aneurysm and it is necessary for an aneurysm repair or graft insertion, a separate CPT code is not reported for the thromboendarterctomy. If only a bypass is placed (requiring an endarterectomy to accomplish), only the bypass is coded. If both an aneurysm repair and a bypass are performed at separate sites, both CPT codes may be assigned, but modifier -59 should be appended to denote a separate procedure on the second code.

When an open vascular procedure such as a thromboendarterectomy is performed, the closure and repair are included in the code for the vascular procedure. CPT codes 35201-35286, which are for reporting repair of blood vessels, are not appropriate to report in addition to a primary vascular procedure for this reason. Also, when a percutaneous vascular procedure is unsuccessful and is followed by an open procedure during the same operative session, only the CPT code for the open procedure should be reported. If the percutaneous procedure was performed for a lesion at one site and the open procedure is performed for a procedure at another site, then separate reporting would be appropriate. Modifier -59 will be used to indicate the separate and distinct nature of the second reported procedure.

Venous access procedure codes 36000, 36406, 36410, and 36415 are used for phlebotomy, prophylactic intravenous access, infusion therapy, chemotherapy drug administration, and other procedures. When intravenous access is performed in the course of performing other medical and surgical procedures or is necessary to accomplish the procedure such as infusion therapy, it is inappropriate to code the access in addition to the greater procedure, since the venous access is integral to the other code. In the case of transcatheter therapy services (i.e., codes 36201, 36202), the placement of the needle and the catheter are included in the primary service. When existing vascular access lines are used to procure arterial or venous blood samples, coding for the sample collection using a separate CPT code is also inappropriate.

Coding Catheters and Infusion Pumps

Some of the most complex coding in the Cardiovascular section is for infusion pumps and catheters for chemotherapy, dialysis, and pain management. The type of device must be identified correctly for appropriate coding. Infusion pumps deliver medication for managing chronic and/or postoperative pain or to administer chemotherapy on a specific time schedule. When the infusion pump reservoir runs out, the patient returns for maintenance and/or refill.

Venous Access Ports

Central venous catheters

Central venous catheters are commonly inserted via the subclavian, jugular, cephalic, femoral, or umbilical veins. Common central venous catheter brand names include Broviac (often used in pediatrics), Hickman, Groshong, and Port-A-Cath. Except for the Broviac and Hickman catheters, all catheters and reservoirs are tunneled just under the skin. Central venous catheters do not have reservoirs and are coded to 36488 or 36489 as appropriate. According to the AMA, a separate code is not reported for the removal of a central venous catheter, as this service would be included in the Evaluation and Management service code for physician services. If the catheter is embedded and requires more than simple suture removal to extricate, then an unlisted code (37799) may be reported with supporting documentation. In the case of a surgical procedure where incision is made for catheter removal, the hospital would assign the appropriate code for the incision.

Infusion pumps

Infusion pumps may be used intravenously (36530-36535) or intra-arterially (36260-36262). For coding, it is essential to confirm which type of pump is employed and the difference between an infusion pump and a venous access port. One type of implantable infusion pump is a disc-like device with two chambers including a side port and a catheter. One chamber contains the material to be infused and the other chamber is called the charging chamber. The charging chamber contains a fluid that expands at body temperature and exerts pressure on the bellows of the pump, forcing the fluid into the catheter. The side port provides access for bolus injections, perfusion studies, or to flush the catheter during routine maintenance. The pump is refilled and bolus injections are administered by use of a Huber needle.

Another type of infusion pump is powered by a lithium battery. This type has a refillable reservoir, an electronic control module, and a miniature peristaltic pump. This type of pump can be programmed using a device outside the body, permitting changes in dosing after the device is implanted. Removal of an implanted intra-arterial infusion pump is coded 36262 and removal of venous access port and/or subcutaneous reservoir is coded 36535.

Other Vascular Procedures

Transluminal angioplasties

The transluminal angioplasties, like cardiac catheterizations, include introduction, positioning and repositioning of the catheters, procurement of blood samples, pressure recordings, and other manipulations required to accomplish the procedure, so assigning a separate code for these services is inappropriate.

Peripheral vascular bypass CPT codes describe bypass procedures using venous grafts (designated by CPT codes 35501-35587) and using other types of bypass procedures such as arterial reconstruction. At a given site of reconstruction, only one type of bypass is performed, so the groups of codes are mutually exclusive. When different sites are treated with different bypass procedures within the same operative session, then the CPT codes for both procedures may be reported, but modifier -59 should be appended to designate the second procedure as distinct from the first.

HEMIC AND LYMPHATIC SYSTEMS

Stem cell harvesting and transplantation

CPT codes are available for procedures performed on the spleen, bone marrow, and lymphatic systems. The codes for stem cell harvesting and transplantation are found in codes 38231, 38240, and 38241. Blood-derived stem cell transplantation differs from bone marrow transplantation, with respect to the source of the transplanted stem cells. In bone marrow transplant, the stem cells are harvested from the patient's bone marrow (autologous) or from a suitable donor (allogenic). In blood-derived stem cell transplant, the cells are acquired from the peripheral blood of the patient or a suitable donor, by one or more apheresis procedures. Over a 1–2 week period, a physician typically performs several 2- to 4-hour apheresis procedures (inpatient or outpatient), which are coded and reported using:

- CPT code 38231 to report the stem cell harvesting, whether performed on the patient or a donor; and
- CPT code 38231 to report "per collection."

It would not be correct to report the therapeutic phlebotomy code 99195 since blood collection is an integral part of stem cell cytopheresis.

For harvesting of a bone marrow specimen, code 85095 is reported and code 86915 describes modification, treatment, and processing of bone marrow specimens for transplantation. For collection of blood specimens, treatment and processing of autologous blood specimens for transplantation use 86890, 86985.

Bone marrow specimens

Code 36520 is used for apheresis procedures related to the management of diseases other than those requiring stem cell transplantation, such as sickle cell disease. This code is also used for reporting plasma apheresis (plasmapheresis) used for the removal of poisons or drugs in acute toxic conditions.

Apheresis procedures

Deep cervical lymph node biopsy or excision (38510) requires an approach through the platysmal muscle. Simple excision of cystic hygroma involves the excision of a hygroma up to 4 cm in size (38550). Complex excision of cystic hygroma involves the excision of a hygroma more than 4 cm in size and deep neurovascular dissection (39555).

Deep cervical lymph node biopsy or excision

DIGESTIVE SYSTEM

CPT coding in the Digestive System section requires an understanding of endoscopy coding. Due to the nature of the digestive tract, many diagnostic and therapeutic procedures may be accomplished by endoscopic approach rather than invasive techniques such as open surgery. Endoscopic services are provided in a variety of facility settings, including a physician's office, ambulatory surgery center, and both hospital inpatient and outpatient departments. Services integral to the endoscopic services such as venous access, noninvasive oximetry, etc., are included in the endoscopy code and are not reported separately for reimbursement. There is a code for anesthesia (often conscious sedation) provided by the surgeon (CPT codes 99141-99142), which is reportable in CPT, but may not always be reimbursed by third party payers. This code requires the presence of a trained observer to assist the physician in monitoring the patient's level of consciousness and physiological status. Medicare carriers do not allow extra reimbursement for this code.

Conscious sedation

When a diagnostic endoscopy is performed in conjunction with a surgical endoscopy, the CPT code selected is the procedure that is the most comprehensive. If a therapeutic service performed repeatedly in the same area, such as may occur in polyp removal, only one code is billed and only one unit of service is indicated on a HCFA 1500 claim form. If different therapeutic services are performed which are not adequately described by the comprehensive code, then additional codes are assigned with Modifier -51. If a diagnostic endoscopy is followed by a surgical endoscopy and/or an open procedure, the diagnostic endoscopy is considered integral to the more comprehensive procedure and is not separately reported.

Gastroenterologic tests included in CPT codes 91000-91299 are frequently complementary to endoscopic procedures. Examples include esophageal and gastric washings for cytology study obtained during an EGD (Esophagastroduodenoscopy or "Upper GI"). When a small intestinal endoscopy is performed as a necessary part of a surgical procedure, the endoscopy is not separately coded. Only in those cases where the endoscopy was

Gastroenterologic tests

performed and a decision to perform further surgery was made based on that endoscopy would an additional code be warranted.

HCFA has developed some specific guidelines for reporting endoscopic biopsies for Medicare outpatients. The term "excision" used in these guidelines includes the variety of terms in the CPT manual that describe the excision or destruction of a lesion (e.g., resection, removal, or fulguration).

HCFA's Guidelines:

1. If a single lesion is biopsied, but not excised, use only the biopsy code.
2. If a biopsy or lesion is obtained and the remaining portion of the same lesion is then excised, code only for the excision.
3. If multiple biopsies are obtained (from the same or different lesions) and none of the lesions is excised, use only the biopsy code and list it once.
4. If a biopsy and an excision are performed, use both codes when the biopsy is taken from a different lesion than the one excised, and the code for the excision does not include the phrase "with or without biopsy." If such a phrase is included, do not use a separate code.

Esophageal dilation

When an endoscopic esophageal dilation is performed, codes 43220-43226 should be selected. Codes 43450-43458 are used only when the dilation is not performed through the endoscope. When dilation fails by unguided sounds and is successfully accomplished by endoscope in the same session, only the more comprehensive procedure should be reported.

When it is necessary to perform a diagnostic endoscopy of the hepatic/pancreatic/biliary system using separate approaches, a CPT code for each approach may be reported. Modifier -51 should be appended to the second procedure code.

Sigmoidoscopy
Colonoscopy

Only the most extensive endoscopic procedure accomplished is reported for a given encounter. For example if a sigmoidoscopy (46330) is completed and a physician performs a colonoscopy (45378) during the same session, only the colonoscopy code is reported. In a colonoscopy, the entire colon, from the rectum to the cecum, is examined.

> *Only the most extensive endoscopic procedure accomplished is reported for a given encounter.*

The examination must include the proximal colon to the splenic flexure, and it may include the terminal ileum.

Endoscopy procedures

Medicare has special reimbursement rules for endoscopy procedures under the RBRVS methodology. If a patient has a colonoscopy and has a polyp removed by snare in one location (45385) and then has a different tumor excised from a different site by hot biopsy forceps (45383), both procedures would be coded. Each of the codes listed includes the base value of the diagnostic colonoscopy code 45378. The procedure with the highest RBRVS total RVUs should be listed first, as it will be reimbursed at 100 percent of the allowed Medicare amount. The lesser valued code will be paid at the full Medicare allowance *minus* the cost of the diagnostic procedure's RVUs. Modifier -59 may be appended to the second procedure to communicate the difference in lesion sites and types.

Exploratory laparotomy
Appendectomy done at time of other major procedure

When open abdominal procedures are performed, the exploration of the surgical field such as the exploratory laparotomy (49000) would not be coded in addition to other more definitive surgery carried out. Appendectomies, for example, are commonly performed incidental to other abdominal procedures. When performed incident to another procedure, the appendectomy should not be coded separately. If performed for an indicated purpose (medically necessary) at the time of another major procedure, then code 44955 is assigned.

Hernia Repair

In CPT, hernia repair codes are categorized primarily by the type of hernia involved. Some types are further specified as to "initial" or "recurrent," based on whether the hernia has required previous repair. Additional variables include patient age and whether the hernia is reducible, incarcerated, or strangulated.

Code 49568 (implantation of mesh or other prosthesis for incisional hernia repair) is used separately when appropriate, or with codes 49560, 49561, 49565, and 49566. It is now possible to repair hernias by use of the laparoscope. For endoscopic repair of inguinal hernia use codes 56315-56317.

Implantation of prosthesis for incisional hernia repair

Endoscopic repair of inguinal hernia

Other Procedures

Additional codes are provided for suturing required for evisceration or dehiscence of an operative incision. There are also codes for omental flaps for reconstruction of sternal and chest wall defects. Code 49905 is an add-on code reported in addition to the code for the primary procedure. When microvascular anastomosis is used code 49906 is assigned.

Procedures performed on the abdomen, omentum, and peritoneum not otherwise listed in CPT may be reported using the unlisted procedure code 49999. As with all reporting of unlisted procedure CPT codes, a copy of the procedure report should be submitted with any third party insurance claim.

Evisceration or dehiscence of operative incision

URINARY SYSTEM

The nature of the urinary system also employs the use of endoscopy in addition to surgical techniques using incisional methods. Many procedures involving the male and female urinary system include the placement of a urethral catheter for postoperative urine drainage. Because insertion of this catheter is integral to the more comprehensive procedure, the catheterization code (53670 and 53675) is not separately coded when performed at the time of or just prior to the surgery. This is true for both physician and hospital reporting. Irrigation and drainage procedures are not generally reported separately when they are integral to successful completion of a more comprehensive operation. Only the code for the comprehensive procedure is assigned. Repair and closure of surgical procedures are also included in the code for the primary procedure. Hernia repair is often included in the code for the service and would not be separately reported, unless the hernia repair and the urinary system procedure involve separate sites. In this case, the secondary procedures will have the -59 modifier appended for the separate site.

Catheterization code

Procedures such as bladder irrigation (51700) performed as a part of a more comprehensive procedure do not merit separate reporting. This code is for irrigation with therapeutic agents when performed independently of surgery. When urethral catheterization or urethral dilation (e.g., codes 53600-53675) are necessary to accomplish another procedure, the urethral catheterization/dilation is not reported in addition to the primary procedure.

Bladder irrigation

Urethral catheterization or dilation

When an endoscopic procedure is performed as an integral part of an open procedure, only the code for the open procedure is reported. Medicare applies the same multiple endoscopy rules to urinary procedures, as was explained above for the digestive system. When several procedures are performed at the same endoscopic session, modifier -51 will be used on the subsequent procedures and adjustments will be made according to HCFA rules for multiple endoscopies.

CPT codes 53502-53515 describe urethral repair codes for urethral wounds or injuries (urethrorrhaphy). When a urethroplasty is performed, codes for urethrorrhaphy should

Urethral repair

not be billed in addition as "suture to repair wound. . .," since this service is included in the urethroplasty service.

Lipoma of spermatic cord

A separate code is not indicated for an excision of a lipoma of spermatic cord (55520) when performed along with an inguinal hernia repair. This incidental removal of a benign neoplasm (lipoma) should not be reported separately for reimbursement.

MALE GENITAL SYSTEM

Needle biopsy of prostate
Ultrasonic guidance

Transrectal ultrasound

Transurethral drainage of prostatic abscess

Biopsy of the prostate is often performed by needles using ultrasonic guidance. To completely code these procedures, one code from the surgery section is used (55700) with an additional code to report the ultrasonic guidance procedure (76942). To report a separate diagnostic ultrasound transrectal procedure in addition to a biopsy with ultrasonic guidance, three codes must be assigned. Code 55700 is reported for the needle biopsy of the prostate, code 76872 is assigned for the transrectal ultrasound, and code 76942 is assigned for the ultrasonic guidance for the prostate biopsy. Because the intent of these ultrasound procedures is different, they are appropriately reported as separate procedures. For hospital coding, these codes are often Charge Master-assigned in the radiology department. For accurate reimbursement and coding, the process of code assignment combining Charge Master-assigned codes and coder-assigned codes should be reviewed carefully. In the APC system, use of both types of codes is likely to impact hospital payment, so the combination of codes and the resulting APC should be evaluated by the coder before submission for payment.

Transurethral drainage of prostatic abscess (e.g., code 52700) is not separately reported in conjunction with more comprehensive prostate procedures. Urethral catheterization is also not coded when performed to accomplish another more complex procedure.

INTERSEX SURGERY

There are codes that exist to report intersex surgery, both changing a male to a female (55870) and a female to a male (55980). These procedures will likely not be reimbursed by health plans unless medical necessity is established. Additional procedure codes may be found in additional sections of CPT depending on the extent and type of surgery that was performed.

LAPAROSCOPY AND HYSTEROSCOPY

Laparoscopy procedures are not restricted to female patients, despite the reference to hysteroscopy in the title of this section. Surgical endoscopy procedures always include the diagnostic portion of the exam so a diagnostic laparoscopy/peritonoscopy/hysteroscopy should be reported only in the absence of further surgery using the endoscope.

When an endoscopic procedure is converted to an open procedure, HCFA guidelines state that only the open procedure be coded and reported. A special ICD-9-CM code (V64.4) is available to explain these circumstances.

Operative laparoscopy and hysteroscopy may employ several methods to accomplish the same

> *When an endoscopic procedure is converted to an open procedure, HCFA guidelines state that only the open procedure be coded and reported. A special ICD-9-CM code (V64.4) is available to explain these circumstances.*

result (e.g., hot cautery, CO2 laser, ND-YAG laser, pelvioscopy), which does not affect the code assignment. When the laparoscopy requires mini-laparotomy (Hasson technique), or requires significantly more time and effort than usual, modifier -22 may be added. Minor procedures such as lysis of adhesions and fulguration of bleeding points are not separately coded.

Any surgery that employs the use of a laparoscope which does not have an existing CPT code assignment in its respective section should be assigned code 56399 (Unlisted procedure, laparoscopy, hysteroscopy), rather than any other unlisted procedure code.

Unlisted procedure, laparoscopy, hysteroscopy

Codes 56343 (salpingostomy) and 56344 (fimbrioplasty) are considered unilateral procedures. When these procedures are performed bilaterally, the modifier -50 should be appended.

Salpingostomy
Fimbrioplasty

FEMALE GENITAL SYSTEM

CPT procedures that use a pelvic examination in conjunction with a gynecologic procedure should not have the pelvic exam coded separately. A diagnostic pelvic exam performed to establish the need and decision for service would be included in the Evaluation and Management service for physicians and is incidental to more comprehensive surgery for hospital reporting. Pelvic examination under anesthesia code 57410 is considered to be included with all major and most minor gynecological procedures for reimbursement purposes, and generally does not warrant separate coding and reporting since it is performed as a routine evaluation of the surgical field.

Pelvic examination under anesthesia

Dilation of the vagina or cervix (e.g., codes 57400-57800), when performed as an approach for female genital system procedures, is not coded separately unless the CPT description states that the more complex procedure is "without cervical dilation."

Dilation of the vagina or cervix

Vulvectomy codes 56620-56640 have specific definitions to follow per the CPT manual:

Vulvectomy

- A *simple procedure* is the removal of skin and superficial subcutaneous tissues.
- A *radical procedure* is the removal of skin and deep subcutaneous tissue.
- A *partial procedure* is the removal of less than 80% of the vulvar area.
- A *complete procedure* is the removal of greater than 80% of the vulvar area.

MATERNITY CARE AND DELIVERY

The codes in section 59000-59899 include only the activities listed in the code descriptions. Additional procedures performed on the same date of service are reported separately with a few exceptions:

- CPT code 59050 (fetal monitoring during labor), code 59300 (episiotomy), and code 59414 (delivery of placenta) are included in the codes for routine obstetric care and do not warrant separate reporting. The consulting physician may use code 59050 to report services. Many health plans use a global package concept for reporting maternity services. What is included in this global package may vary from payer to payer. Not included in the global services are ultrasound procedures, amniocentesis, special screening for genetic conditions, visit code for unrelated conditions, or additional visits and services for high risk conditions or complications.

Fetal monitoring during labor
Episiotomy
Delivery of placenta

- Specific codes (59610-59622) are assigned for women who present for delivery following a previous Cesarean section. The appropriate code for vaginal delivery after previous Cesarean delivery is 59610, including the routine antepartum and postpartum care, or code 59612 or 59614, for components of it.

Delivery following a previous Cesarean section
Vaginal delivery

- Cesarean delivery after an attempted vaginal delivery (history of previous C-section) has a special range of codes (59618-59622) available for this situation.

Cesarean delivery

Maternity care   Those situations where different physicians are involved with maternity care can make code selection more complex. For example, often a family practice physician takes care of routine vaginal deliveries but refers Cesarean section births to a surgeon or OB/GYN specialist. When a patient requires a Cesarean section, another physician is called upon to operate, with the family practice physician assisting. To appropriately code that situation, we assume that the family physician saw the patient more than seven times and resumes postpartum care after delivery. This physician reports codes 59426, 59414-80, and 59430 to show that antepartum care, assistance at C-section, and postpartum care were all provided. Selected insurance plans may have the physician report 59510 with the -80 modifier appended as a global fee.

ENDOCRINE AND NERVOUS SYSTEM

Intracranial surgery   A burr hole is often required for intracranial surgery such as craniotomy and craniectomy. This procedure along with taps, punctures, or other drainage procedures followed by more extensive surgery would not be separately coded. Many of the intracranial procedures include bone grafting within the CPT definition and would not require a separate code for the bone graft. Biopsies performed in the course of more comprehensive surgery are also not coded separately, and neither are exploratory surgery codes 61304-61305 when another procedure is performed at the same session. The use of intravascular access devices, cardiac monitoring, oximetry, and other monitoring would not merit separate coding when performed in conjunction with a CNS procedure.

Excision of lesions involving the skull base may require the skills of several surgeons with different surgical specialties working together at the same time. These procedures are categorized into the approach procedure, the definitive procedure (biopsy, lesion removal, etc.), and the repair or reconstruction procedure. Each surgeon involved in these cases reports only the CPT codes for the specific procedure personally performed. If one surgeon performs more than one procedure, then modifier -51 is appended to the secondary, additional procedure(s).

When a spinal puncture is performed, the local anesthesia necessary to perform the spinal puncture is included in the procedure itself.

Paravertebral facet injections   Paravertebral facet injections are coded using CPT codes 64440✻, 64441✻, 64442✻, and 64443✻, depending on location and number of levels injected. Each lumbar joint is innervated by two nerves. When paravertebral facet joints are blocked (two facets, right and left at a single level) code 64442 is reported. Whether the paravertebral facet nerve root injection is considered unilateral or bilateral is dependent on the technique used. Imaging and fluoroscopy services are not included in the joint nerve injection codes and

Imaging and fluoroscopy   would have a separate code from the 70000-76000 series reported in addition to the injection along with CPT code 99070 or the appropriate HCPCS for the provision of the radiopharmaceutical agent used for imaging.

Injection of steroids   It should be noted that these injection codes are for anesthetic agents. CPT does not currently have codes for injection of other substances (e.g., steroids) into the facet joints. Injections may be predominantly anesthetic or steroids, depending on the source of pain. In the case of steroid injection, *CPT Assistant* (Vol. 6, No. 4, April 1996) recommends use of the unlisted procedure code 64999 with documentation describing what was done to any third party payer involved (see "Coding a Facet Joint Injection," *CPT Assistant*, Vol. 6, No. 4, April 1996, pp. 6–7).

Epidural injections   Epidural injections for pain management or anesthesia are found in the Injection, Drainage, or Aspiration section of CPT. When the substance injected is predominantly anesthetic or antispasmodic, codes 62274-62279 are assigned. Injection of neurolytic substances is included in the range of 62280-62282. Injection of other materials (i.e., steroids) is reported using CPT code 62289.

EYE AND OCULAR ADNEXA

Procedures involving the eyeball, anterior segment, posterior segment, and other ocular adnexa are found in the code range 67112-67299. This section of CPT is primarily used to report the services of ophthalmologists or for hospital reporting of outpatient surgery involving the eyes.

When exenteration of the orbit (65110, 65112, 65114) is performed, assign a separate code for the skin grafting from codes 15120, 15121, 15260, or 15261.

Evisceration (65091, 65093) is a partial enucleation wherein the scleral shell is left intact while the intraocular contents are removed.

Cataract procedures are very common in the Medicare population. For coding purposes, the following procedure(s) performed with cataract extraction are not to be separately coded:

Cataract procedures

- anterior capsulotmy
- enzymatic zonulysis
- iridectomy
- iridotomy
- lateral canthotomy
- pharmacological agents used
- posterior capsulotomy
- subconjunctival and subtenon injections
- viscoelastic agents

Cataract extractions are always coded based on the type of procedure performed:

- Intracapsular cataract extraction (ICCE) is the surgical removal of the entire lens, with the lens capsule (front and back) intact.
- Extracapsular cataract extraction is the surgical removal of the front portion and the nucleus of the lens leaving the posterior capsule in place. Endocapsular extraction is the same procedure.
- Phacofragmentation describes the breaking of the lens into fragments by mechanical means, usually ultrasound. Phacoemulsification describes the breaking of the lens into tiny particles by ultrasonic waves which are suctioned out after fragmentation.

Cataract extraction codes 66983 and 66984 include the insertion of the intraocular lens prosthesis. In the APC system for hospital and ASC reimbursement, the payment for the lens is included in the APC amount for Medicare patients and is not reported separately.

Cataracts do not recur after removal, but it is common for a secondary cataract, often referred to as an "after-cataract" (secondary membrane or opacification of capsule) to form as a result of clouding of the capsule behind the intraocular lens. This condition is treated with a Neodymium Yttrium Aluminum Garnet laser, commonly referred to as a YAG laser. A laser capsulotomy may be used to create an opening in the capsule to enable light to reach the retina. This procedure is coded in CPT using 66821.

After-cataract

Strabismus surgery on the extraocular muscles of the eye may be indicated if nonsurgical means fail to adequately control misalignment of the eyes. These procedures are coded in the range of 67311-67340. There are two horizontal muscles (lateral rectus and medial rectus) in each eye and four vertical muscles (superior and inferior rectus muscles and the superior and inferior oblique muscles). To correctly code strabismus procedures the number and position of the muscles involved must be verified with the operative report. The CPT codes for strabismus refer to each eye separately. If the same operation is performed for both eyes, the modifier for bilateral procedures (-50) is appended to the code. If horizontal and vertical procedures are both performed, more than one code will be

Strabismus surgery

needed to report the procedure. The add-on codes 67331 and 67332 refer to extensive operations on the eyes previously operated on. Re-operation procedures require more skill and effort, and so have higher RVU values than the codes for initial strabismus surgery. According to the AMA, the parenthetical note which says "patient not previously operated on" in codes 67311-67318 in CPT 1998 does not preclude use of these codes for subsequent strabismus surgery. This reference was dropped in 1999.

Codes 67320, 67331, 67332, 67335, and 67340 are considered add-on codes. The basic procedure is reported using the appropriate surgery code (CPT codes 67311-67318) and these add-on codes are also reported to describe circumstances specific to the case. For example, if two horizontal muscles in a patient's left eye require surgery use code 67312. These muscles were previously operated on, so code 67332 is added. The patient also has one vertical muscle of the right eye operated on during this session (code 67314). This muscle was operated on previously, so code 67332 is also reported again. For this case, a total of four codes—67312, 67332, 67314-51, and 67332—would be listed on a HCFA 1500 or UB-92 (no -51 modifier would be used for hospital coding). When the third party payer accepts HCPCS Level II modifiers, the HCPCS modifiers RT and LT (left and right) for reporting may be helpful to show that the repeated code is for the other eye.

When a subconjunctival injection (e.g., code 68200) with a local anesthetic is performed as part of a more extensive anesthesia procedure for eye surgery, it is not appropriate to code it separately. Also iridectomy, trabeculectomy, and anterior vitrectomy may be performed in conjunction with cataract removal when an iridectomy is performed to accomplish a cataract extraction. A trabeculectomy performed to control glaucoma at the same time as a cataract extraction may be separately coded with the different diagnosis. A trabeculectomy performed as a preventive service for an expected transient increase in intraocular pressure postoperatively without other evidence of glaucoma would not warrant separate coding.

Repairs of brow ptosis, blepharoptosis, or lid retraction

CPT codes 67900-67924 (for repairs of brow ptosis, blepharoptosis, or lid retraction) include CPT codes for blepharoplasty (15820-15823) as part of the total service. Canthoplasty code 67950 is included in repair procedures such as blepharoplasties. Ectropion/entropion (codes 67917 and 67924) include the blepharoplasty procedures that may be needed to complete the major procedure on the same eyelid so the blepharoplasty codes would not be necessary.

Incision and drainage of the conjunctiva

Codes for incision and drainage of the conjunctiva (68020-68200) are included in all conjunctivoplasties (68320-68362). Correction of lid retraction code 67911 includes the full thickness skin graft code 15260, so both codes would not be reported together.

The injection code(s) for sclerosing agents in the same session as glaucoma surgery are not separately coded.

Eyelid procedures

Eyelid procedures for removal of lesions and blepharoplasty procedures always include more than skin. If lid margin, tarsus, and/or palpebral conjunctiva are not involved, the procedures should be coded using integumentary system code(s) 11440-11446 or 11640-11646. Codes 17000-17004 are used for lesion removal, or there are appropriate codes for repair.

Corneal transplant codes

Corneal transplant codes 65710-65755 include the use of fresh or preserved grafts and preparation of donor material. An additional HCPCS code V2785 is available for Medicare patients for processing, preserving, and transporting corneal tissue. The codes for penetrating keratoplasty include a diagnosis within the descriptions so a careful review of the medical record documentation is required before selecting a procedure code.

Repetitive services for prophylaxis or destruction of retinal conditions include "one or more sessions" in the descriptions for codes 67141-67228. When these codes are reported they are not repeated for subsequent encounters for repeated treatments.

AUDITORY SYSTEM

Diagnostic services such as audiometry and vestibular testing are found in the Medicine section of CPT. The surgical section for auditory systems encompasses codes 69000-69979, which are used to report procedures involving the ear.

When a mastoidectomy is included in the description of another auditory procedure the separate code for a mastoidectomy is not reported.

When insertion of a ventilating tube is performed with myringotomy, codes 69420 or 69421 are not appropriate since codes 69433 or 69436 will be assigned. Removal of a ventilating tube (69424) is not reported by the same physician who inserted it, since it is considered part of routine follow-up. For hospital reporting, removal of the tube likely does not warrant separate coding when performed in the course of another procedure, such as replacement of the tube.

Audiometry and vestibular testing

Mastoidectomy

Myringotomy with tube insertion

RADIOLOGY CODING GUIDELINES: CODES 70010-79999

In the Radiology section of CPT there are several notes preceding certain subsections that are important for coders to understand. In radiology, it is common for a procedure to have both professional and technical components. When a procedure is performed by two physicians, the radiologic portion of the procedure is designated as "radiological supervision and interpretation." When a physician performs both the procedure and in addition provides imaging supervision and interpretation, then a combination of codes from the Surgery section and the 70000 series of codes will be required for complete reporting. Supervision and interpretation codes will not apply to the section for Radiation Oncology. Written reports signed by the interpreting physician should be considered an integral part of a radiologic procedure or interpretation. Most health plans would not provide reimbursement to a provider who billed for interpretation services without completion of a formal written report of findings.

Noninvasive, noninterventional diagnostic imaging includes standard X-rays in single or multiple views, contrast studies, computerized tomography (CAT scans) and magnetic resonance imaging (MRI). Since there are a number of CPT coding options it is important to determine the most comprehensive code rather than reporting multiple codes for each individual view. In the event that radiographs must be repeated in the course of an encounter due to substandard quality, only one code should be reported for the service for payment purposes. When more extensive radiographs are required after the initial service, the code for the comprehensive service should be reported, even when the patient has to return to the radiology suite for the extended examination.

When limited comparative radiographs are performed for post-fracture reduction, post-intubation, post-catheter placement, etc., it is appropriate for physicians to use the -52 modifier for reduced interpretive services.

Radiologic studies may be performed without contrast, with contrast, or both with and without contrast. There are special codes to describe these services which include all radiographs necessary to complete the study. Unless specifically noted, fluoroscopy necessary to complete a procedure and obtain the necessary permanent radiographic record is included in the major procedure performed and is not separately reported.

When contrast is administered orally or rectally, the administration is included as part of the CPT code for the service. When the contrast media has to be injected, the administration and the injection are included in the contrast studies CPT code. When a contrast study is performed in which there is direct correlation of the timing of the study to the injection or administration such as angiography, and different physicians perform separate parts of the procedure, each physician would report the service personally rendered. The procedural aspect of the service will come from the Surgery section in CPT and then the supervision and interpretation will be selected from the Radiology section. Hospitals will also report both codes to reflect the complete procedure. The codes in the Radiology section will indicate which injection codes to report. When no parenthetical note appears an additional code would not be assigned. For example, a placement of an intravenous line placed for access only is considered part of the procedure and does not warrant separate coding.

Arterial catheterization

For selective vascular catheterization, the codes include introduction of the catheter and all lesser order selective catheterizations used in the approach. Additional second and/or third order arterial catheterizations within the same family of arteries supplied by a single first order artery are expressed using CPT code 36218 or 36248, according to the notes in the Aorta and Arteries subsection in the Radiology section of CPT. The procedure codes and the radiology codes for selective vascular catheterization are reported separately, as there is no CPT code for the complete procedure.

Diagnostic ultrasound procedures have the following definitions listed in CPT:

- **A-mode** implies a one-dimensional ultrasonic measurement procedure.
- **M-mode** implies a one-dimensional ultrasonic measurement procedure with movement of the trace to record amplitude and velocity of moving echo-producing structures.
- **B-scan** implies a two-dimensional ultrasonic scanning procedure with a two-dimensional display.
- **Real-time scan** implies a two-dimensional ultrasonic scanning procedure with display of both two-dimensional structure and motion with time.

Specific guidelines for use of the Radiation Oncology services are listed in the CPT manual in this subsection.

Imaging studies

Within the Cardiovascular System in the Radiology Section, myocardial perfusion and cardiac imaging studies may be performed at rest and/or during stress. When performed during exercise and/or pharmacologic stress, the appropriate stress testing code from the 93015-93018 series should be reported in addition to code(s) 78460, 78465, 78472, 78473, 78481, and 78483.

PATHOLOGY AND LABORATORY GUIDELINES FOR CODES 80049-89999

The Pathology and Laboratory section of CPT includes services directed at evaluation of specimens from the patient's body fluids, tissues, and cell samples to provide information to the treating physician. Consideration of this evaluation, combined with the medical history and physical examination findings, provide a basis for medical decision making. Generally, many of the laboratory procedures are prepared and/or screened by laboratory technicians with a pathologist reviewing the product and assuming responsibility for the integrity of the results generated by the laboratory. This is why this section of CPT contains very few codes to reflect patient contact. If a pathologist does provide separately identifiable services, they would be coded in the Evaluation and Management section of CPT.

Hospitals and independent laboratories are heavy users of this section of CPT. Physicians and clinics also report selected procedures from this section. With the inclusion of many laboratory tests into disease and/or organ panels it is important for codes to be selected within panels when appropriate rather than "unbundling" a panel of tests into individual ones reported separately. The tests listed within each panel identify the components of the panel reported. Organization of specified tests into panels does not preclude the separate reporting of additional tests not included in the panel when performed for a specific purpose. Third party payers become concerned when no order for a specific test is recorded, yet reimbursement is sought from a lab or hospital for a separate test that the physician believed to be part of a panel.

Surgical pathology codes (CPT codes 88300-88309) include accession, examination, and reporting of pathological specimens obtained in surgery. CPT defines a specimen as tissue or tissue(s) that are submitted for individual and separate attention, requiring individual examination and pathologic diagnosis. There are six levels of service beginning with gross examination only at Level I and progressing through ascending levels of physician work to complex gross and microscopic examination in Level VI. Any unlisted specimen should be assigned to the code that most closely reflects the physician work involved when compared to other specimens assigned to that code.

Surgical pathology

For physician reporting of laboratory procedures within their offices, the Clinical Laboratory Improvement Act (CLIA) has strengthened oversight requirements and allows only selected procedures to be performed without meeting stringent regulatory requirements. A list of CLIA-waived tests is available from the Medicare carrier appropriate to the practice location. A sample of CLIA-waived tests from one carrier in 1998 is available at www.empiremedicare.com/benenews/brf984/clia.htm.

MEDICINE SECTION GUIDELINES

The Medicine section of CPT contains both diagnostic and therapeutic services performed by physicians and some other health care professionals. Before Evaluation and Management codes were provided in 1992, visit codes for physician services were located in this section of CPT. This part of CPT contains codes for noninvasive or minimally invasive services that are not considered either surgical or Evaluation and Management in nature.

Immunization injections are normally provided in the course of an evaluation and management service. The code for the injection includes the supply of materials injected and the administration of the injection, although some third party payers provide separate reimbursement for each component. For example, in 1998, Medicare provided reimbursement for influenza injections when CPT code 90724 was reported. Additional reimbursement is provided for the administration of the flu shot by reporting a separate HCPCS code G0008, which for other payers is included in the 90724 code. CPT instructions state that if the immunization is not provided in the course of another service, the minimal service code (99211) may be assigned. In 1999, new codes for the administration of immunizations were provided.

Immunization injections

Codes for other therapeutic or diagnostic infusions and injections do not include the supply of the injected materials. These should be added by reporting the appropriate "J" code in HCPCS or using the 99070 code for supplies provided in CPT, depending on the instructions of the insurance carrier where payment is sought. Medicare considers the administration of an injection bundled into the Evaluation and Management services provided at the same time, and other health plans may also follow this rule.

Infusions and injections

Chemotherapy injections have their own section (codes 96400-96549) and are independent of the patient's visit services, so may be separately coded. If an Evaluation and Management service is reported, the documentation should reflect significantly identifiable services that include history, examination, and medical decision making in addition to the chemotherapy service. To appropriately code chemotherapy when different techniques are used, separate codes for each parenteral method of administration should be reported. Other medications that are administered independently or sequentially as supportive management of chemotherapy administration should be separately reported using 90780-90788,

Chemotherapy

as appropriate. For Medicare patients, modifier -59 should be added to the injection service to communicate a distinct service. Medicare does not pay for these drugs administered at the same time as chemotherapy, but will reimburse for the service when it is sequential on the same day. The provision of the chemotherapy agent is coded using HCPCS "J" codes for Medicare patients or, for other payers, CPT code 96545 may be reported for the drug.

The APC system reimburses hospitals for outpatient chemotherapy on the basis of the "J" code drug administered by categorizing them into Level I, II, III, or IV, which comprise APC groups 061, 062, 063 and 064, rather than the CPT code.

Psychiatric codes

Psychiatric codes in CPT have specific guidelines for use that must be reviewed before a code is selected for mental health services. Drug management is included in some of the therapeutic services such as CPT codes 90842-90844, 90847, and 90853, so it would not be correct to assign code 90862 in addition to these services.

General Opthalmological Services

The Medicine section includes General Ophthalmological Services in codes 92002-92013. Definitions of the services that constitute an intermediate and comprehensive examination are detailed in the Ophthalmology subsection. The same definitions for new and established patients in the E/M section of CPT apply to the eye examination codes. If a patient has not received any services within 3 years he or she is considered a new patient. If Evaluation and Management codes are used for a single specialty examination, the eye exams cannot be reported in addition to eye exam codes, but must be used instead of them. Either set of codes may be used by the ophthalmologist, since code selection will depend on the nature and purpose of the encounter. The codes in the Special Ophthalmologic Services section represent specific services that are not described as part of a general or routine ophthalmological examination. Gonioscopy (separate procedure), coded 92020, is considered bundled with the eye examination codes for many health insurance carriers, including Medicare. Ophthalmoscopy is part of General and Special Ophthalmologic Services whenever indicated and is not reported separately when carried out in conjunction with them.

Refraction

Medicare Part B fee-for-service does not cover routine eye care, but allows reporting of a separate charge for refraction when other covered services are provided in addition to it. Code 92015 is used for this purpose. The intent of CPT is very clear, that determination of the refractive state is not included in a comprehensive ophthalmology service.

Special guidelines are described in the Special Otorhinolaryngologic subsection, including both diagnostic and therapeutic procedures. These should be reviewed when selecting codes from this area. Audiologic Function Tests with Medical Evaluation codes imply the use of calibrated electronic equipment. Tests normally included in a general otorhinolaryngologic examination would not be coded separately. If a test is conducted on only one ear, modifier -52 should be appended to communicate a reduced service, since CPT assumes that both ears are tested.

The codes in the Cardiovascular Medicine subsection include noninvasive and some invasive diagnostic testing including intracardiac catheterization and percutaneous angioplasty.

Cardiopulmonary resuscitation

When cardiopulmonary resuscitation is performed without other Evaluation and Management services rendered to the patient such as Critical Care, only the code for the CPR (92950) should be reported. A typical circumstance has a physician directing a "code blue" situation, with the patient's attending physician taking over following the successful CPR session. The time required to perform CPR is not included in critical care codes or other Evaluation and Management services, so both codes may be reported by a physician when both services are rendered.

A number of therapeutic and diagnostic cardiovascular procedures routinely utilize intravenous or intra-arterial vascular access, require EKG monitoring, and require agents administered either by injection or infusion. Routine services that are integral to the primary procedure would not be separately reported in CPT. In specific circumstances where the procedure is not routinely part of the more comprehensive service, separate reporting may be warranted.

Cardiac catheterization is often an area where code assignment is complex for both physician use and facility reporting. CPT codes relevant to a cardiac catheterization procedure include codes 93501-93536, 93541-93545, and 93555-93556. To accurately report cardiac catheterization, it must be known what is included in the catheterization procedure and when selective injection procedures should be coded. Modifier -51 is not appended to any of the codes in the 93501-93556 range. It is necessary to report all of the procedures required to provide the diagnostic picture when coding a cardiac catheterization procedure. Modifier -26 is appropriately appended only to codes 93501-93536. Codes 93539-93545 and 93555-93556 would not be reported with modifier -26. The codes in the 93555-93556 range are reported only once even though multiple angiographic procedures may have been performed.

Cardiac catheterization

PTCA (Percutaneous Transluminal Coronary Angioplasty) is a less invasive method of treating plaque formation in the coronary arteries than open heart procedures. When coding the angioplasty of a single vessel, code 92982 is used. This code includes the introduction, positioning, and repositioning of the catheter within that single vessel. Any injection of dye and related imaging to determine the catheter/balloon placement and post-procedure effectiveness are included and should not be reported separately. If multiple lesions are treated within a single vessel, the code is still reported only once. If more than one vessel is treated during the same session, code 92984 is assigned in addition to 92982. This is an add-on code that will not stand alone and would not require modifier -51 for multiple procedures. Pre-procedure diagnostic cardiac catheterization, even when performed on the same date as angioplasty, should be separately reported. PTCAs are often performed in the cardiac cath lab with catheterization integral to the procedure. In this situation, separate reporting is not appropriate. Angioplasty of other vessels (non-cardiac) will be coded in the range of 35470-35476.

Percutaneous Transluminal Coronary Angioplasty

Allergy and Clinical Immunology services are reported by selecting codes 95004-95199. Notes within the subsection define allergy sensitivity tests, immunotherapy, and other therapies that are assigned to this section. Evaluation and Management codes are reported in addition to allergy testing or immunology services only when significant, separately identifiable services in addition to the allergy service are provided. The number of percutaneous tests performed in codes 95004, 95010, 95015, 95024, 95028, 95044, and 95052 should be reported in addition to the CPT code in the units field of the HCFA 1500 form. The number of doses should be reported in conjunction with CPT code 95165 and 95170.

Allergy and Clinical Immunology

The Neurology and Neuromuscular Procedure subsection in CPT includes codes for sleep testing, nerve and muscle testing, and electroencephalographic procedures. CPT requirements for sleep testing are detailed in the notes. The EEG, evoke potential, and sleep services codes include the tracing, interpretation, and report. When only the interpretation portion of the service is provided, modifier -26 is used. Separate procedure codes may be assigned for the EEGs provided separate from sleep studies if the EEG is not integral to the sleep study but rather separately performed during another session on the same date of service. Modifier -59 is used on the EEG to indicate that the service is distinct, and when appropriate different ICD-9-CM codes are assigned.

Sleep testing
Nerve and muscle testing
Electroencephalographic procedures

CPT CODING FOR ANCILLARY SERVICES PROVIDED IN HOSPITALS

CPT is now firmly established as a reporting system for hospital outpatient services. Coding outpatient procedures for facility services generally follows the same rules that apply to physician use of codes to report services rendered. One must remember that CPT reporting by a hospital is for the facility portion of the service which may or may not include professional interpretations, depending on the nature of the relationship of the hospital with the interpreting physician. When the hospital provides for both the professional and technical elements of an ancillary service such as a radiology procedure, CPT codes for a complete procedure or codes reported without modification are used.

Typically hospitals automate code assignment for ancillary services by use of a Charge Master system. This may also be called Charge Description Master (CDM) or Service Description Master. This computer program facilitates accurate automated coding of the service at the time it is ordered by the clinician performing the test, rather than code assignment by staff based on the documentation of the service. When the procedure is ordered, the system maps to the correct CPT code for billing, so no analysis of records is required to capture all of the tests performed for a patient. A coding professional typically assigns the ICD-9-CM code only for the claim since the CPT code has already been stored. When the claim is prepared, the human-assigned diagnosis code and computer-generated CPT code from the Charge Master meet on the UB-92 form. Often ancillary procedures are performed in conjunction with surgical procedures, so for hospital outpatient reporting, a CPT code is assigned following analysis of the operative records and the associated ancillary services come in via the Charge Master. In an APG (Ambulatory Payment Groups) and/or APC (Ambulatory Patient Classification) system, both of these sources will be used to establish a prospective payment amount through classification to a specified group. Viewing of the complete set of codes assigned, with a look at the grouping that results in the applicable APC or APG, will be necessary to assure correct payment in these systems. Procedures found in the Medicine section of CPT will have designated APC groups associated with them. Services where time or level of care is designated may have a reimbursement impact in this prospective payment system. Some codes in this section are "bundled" or "packaged" with other codes and do not result in separate payment by reporting.

Surgical Coding Exercises

Assign CPT codes for the following narrative descriptions:

1. Open reduction, nasal fracture, uncomplicated

2. Administration of anesthesia, for breast reduction mammoplasty procedure, normal healthy patient

3. Colectomy, with continent ileostomy

4. Total abdominal hysterectomy; bilateral salpingo-oophorectomy

5. Vaginal delivery with midline episiotomy, "drop in"—no prenatal care or postpartum services rendered

6. Neonate circumcision using clamp

7. Insertion of indwelling ureteral stent by cystourethroscopic approach

8. Endoscopic injection of collagen into the urethra and/or bladder neck for urinary incontinence

9. Split thickness skin graft for extensive partial thickness wounds to the abdomen from previous abdominoplasty for morbid obesity. Size of defect less than 80 sq. cm with excisional preparation of the site performed.

10. Acute coronary artery bypass graft times two with left internal mammary artery to left anterior descending coronary artery and left reverse autogenous saphenous vein graft to the first diagonal branch of the left anterior descending

11. Cystourethroscopy, distal left ureteral dilation and placement of ureteral stent

12. Total endoscopic ethmoidectomy and septoplasty with submucous resection

13. Bronchoscopy with transbronchial needle biopsy

14. Removal common warts (3) using cryotherapy technique

15. Arthroscopy of the knee with medial meniscectomy and meniscal shaving and debridement

16. Arthroscopic removal of loose body, ankle

17. Excision of a total of three chalazion, both eyelids

18. Intracapsular cataract extraction with insertion of lens

19. Tympanoplasty with ossicular chain reconstruction

20. Destruction of penile herpetic lesions by laser

Radiology Coding Exercises

Use the CPT manual and appropriate guidelines to code the following:

1. Radiologists who are not employed by the facility where they practice will most often report:
   a. The CPT codes in the Radiology section that represent complete procedures.
   b. Each CPT code with an HCPCS modifier that indicates technical component of procedures.
   c. CPT codes that represent the supervision and interpretation of radiology procedures.
   d. Codes from the Evaluation and Management section of CPT.

2. The correct code for imaging using PET technology in the brain for metabolic evaluation is:
   a. 78807
   b. 78608
   c. 78800
   d. 78810

3. Clinical Treatment Management in Radiation Therapy is based on _____ fractions delivered comprising one week regardless of the intervals between treatments.
   a. 7
   b. 4
   c. 10
   d. 5

4. The CPT definition of "conformal" in Clinical Treatment Management for Radiation Therapy is:
   a. Three or more separate treatment areas, highly complex blocking, tangential ports, wedges, rational compensators or other special beam considerations.
   b. Multiple custom megavoltage treatment beams focused on a large three dimensional target.
   c. Use of special blocks, two separate treatment areas, three or more ports on a single treatment area.
   d. Single treatment area, single port or parallel opposed ports or simple blocks.

5. Ultrasonic examination in a supervision of high risk multiple pregnancy before the second trimester is coded:
   a. 76700
   b. 76810
   c. 76805
   d. 76815

Pathology and Laboratory Coding Exercises

Use the 1999 CPT manual and appropriate guidelines to code the following:

1. An ACTH stimulation panel for adrenal insufficiency which includes three cortisols is performed in a hospital outpatient laboratory. What CPT code(s) should be found in the Charge Master for this service?
   a. 82530 Cortisol; free
   b. 82533 Cortisol, total
   c. 80400 ACTH stimulation panel; for adrenal insufficiency + 82533
   d. 80412 Corticotropic releasing hormone (CRH) stimulation panel

2. How is a "stat laboratory test" reported in CPT?
   a. There is no mechanism for reporting emergency performed tests in CPT. The code is reported the same as routine laboratory tests.
   b. By coding the specified test and applying a modifier -22 for unusual circumstances.
   c. By choosing the CPT codes that have "immediately performed" in their description.
   d. By using an add-on code for the "stat" portion of the procedure.

3. What is the appropriate CPT code for a placenta reviewed following vaginal delivery for the pathologists' reporting?
   a. 88304 (Level III) Surgical Pathology; gross and microscopic examination
   b. 88307(Level V) Surgical Pathology; gross and microscopic examination
   c. 88305 (Level IV) Surgical Pathology; gross and microscopic examination
   d. 59414 Delivery of the placenta (separate procedure)

4. The CPT code used for a quick test "strep screen" performed in a physician's office for a sore throat is:
   a. 87430 Streptococcus, group A
   b. 86588 Streptococcus screen direct
   c. 87880 Direct Optical Observation
   d. 86403-86408 Particle agglutination screens

5. What code is assigned for reporting a coroner's call following a homicide?
   a. 88040 Necropsy; forensic examination
   b. 88045 Necropsy; coroner's call
   c. 88000 Necropsy (autopsy), gross examination only; without CNS
   d. 88099 Unlisted necropsy (autopsy) procedure

Medicine Coding Exercises

1. When coding injections in CPT using the range of codes 90782-90789, what additional element should be reported that is not reflected in the code?
   a. The office visit should always be coded in addition to this service.
   b. A modifier is required for each of these codes for Medicare reporting.
   c. The material injected must be specified.
   d. The method of administration must be specified.

2. The CPT code for gastric lavage is:
   a. 91055 Gastric intubation
   b. 91052 Gastric analysis test
   c. 91020 Gastric motility studies
   d. 91105 Gastric intubation, and aspiration or lavage for treatment

3. CPT codes for immunizations. . .
   a. should not be coded with an Evaluation and Management service.
   b. require modifiers for Medicare reporting.
   c. include the materials involved in the administration of the immunization.
   d. must be reported with code 99211.

4. Allergy injection code 95115. . .
   a. does not include the provision of the allergenic extracts.
   b. is used for two or more injections of allergenic extracts.
   c. is not reported with an office visit Evaluation and Management code.
   d. requires the addition of a HCPCS Level II code for Medicare reporting.

5. Adjunct codes found in the Special Services and Reports section of CPT are used. . .
   a. for reporting services that are always bundled into other CPT codes.
   b. for reporting services in addition to basic services in CPT, as additional codes.
   c. for chiropractic care.
   d. for services that are never reimbursed by health plans and must be billed to the patient.

6. When codes 90782-90799 are assigned for an injection, what additional reporting should occur that is not included in the code description?
   a. material injected (by narrative description or HCPCS Level II code)
   b. an Evaluation and Management code
   c. method of infusion
   d. chemotherapy drugs

7. How many codes are assigned for a comprehensive eye examination with gonioscopy for a new patient?
   a. Three: one for the eye exam, one for the "visit," and one for the gonioscopy
   b. Two: one for the comprehensive eye exam and the other for new patient exam
   c. One, since gonioscopy is a "separate procedure" included in the comprehensive eye exam
   d. One, because gonioscopy includes the eye exam services

8. A patient presents to a physician's office for a flu shot. According to CPT guidelines, what code(s) may be assigned for services?
   a. 90724 and 99213
   b. 90724 and 99211 or 99025
   c. 90724
   d. 90749 and 99211 or 990259

9. What code would be used when a cardiovascular surgeon performs PTCA of the left anterior descending artery?
   a. 92984
   b. 92980
   c. 92982
   d. 92995

10. An office visit with osteopathic manipulation requires the coder to review the following from the medical record to assign the correct CPT code:
    a. if a separately identifiable service occurred in addition to the manipulative treatment and how many body regions were involved in the manipulation
    b. the time spent in manipulation of the body regions
    c. the reason for the manipulation (ICD-9-CM coded diagnosis)
    d. the health plan paying for the osteopathic manipulation

8 CPT Modifier Usage

The stated purpose of modifier numbers in CPT is to "provide the means by which the reporting physician can indicate that a service or procedure that has been performed has been altered by some specific circumstance but not changed in definition or code" (*CPT 1998* [Chicago: American Medical Association, 1998], p. x). Modifiers have long been available for CPT codes to report physician services. Hospitals were directed to report selected modifiers for Medicare patients in 1998 in preparation for the Ambulatory Payment Classification (APC) system of prospective payment for hospital and Ambulatory Surgery Center outpatients. From a third party payer perspective, CPT or HCPCS modifiers provide additional information needed to process claims more efficiently and with less delay. Some of the modifiers have a direct effect on reimbursement, while others have only an indirect effect by clarifying situations that govern coverage issues.

The 1998 CPT manual lists the following examples of situations that merit modifier reporting. Use modifiers when:

1. A service has both a technical and a professional component (and you want to report only one or the other).
2. A service or procedure was performed by more than one physician and/or in more than one location.
3. A service or procedure has been increased or reduced (from the services listed in the code description).
4. Only part of a service was performed.
5. An adjunctive procedure was performed.
6. A bilateral procedure was performed (and bilaterality is not mentioned in the code description).
7. A service or procedure was performed more than once (and a method is needed to prevent denial as a duplicate service).
8. Unusual events occurred (that did not alter the basic description, but contributed to resource utilization or other factors that impact reporting or reimbursement). (*CPT 1998* [Chicago: American Medical Association, 1998] p. x.)

Appendix A in the back of the CPT manual lists the modifiers available in the current year for use with CPT. It is important to understand that the above list is not a set of conditions where modifiers are always required or even appropriate. For example:

1. Some CPT codes include the technical and professional components. Use of the -26 modifier with these codes is incorrect. For example, code 93000 (Electrocardiogram, routine ECG with at least 12 lead; with interpretation and report) includes both professional and technical components in the code description. Code 71010 (Radiologic examination, chest; single view, frontal) includes both the technical and professional components in the description. To report only the professional component, as would be common for a radiologist, modifier -26 (professional component) must be employed. When an insurance processor sees the -26 modifier on a claim for the chest X-ray the reimbursement will be adjusted since only the professional component of the services is paid to the physician, and the hospital will receive an amount to compensate for technical services only (equipment and technician costs). There is

no modifier in CPT that denotes technical component. The HCPCS Level II modifier -TC is recognized by Medicare, Medicaid, and selected other payers.

2. The situation of a service or procedure being performed by more than one physician or in more than one location may also not always warrant the reporting of a modifier. For example, most health plans do not pay additional amounts for a code such as 67227, Destruction of extensive or progressive retinopathy (e.g., diabetic retinopathy), one or more sessions, cryotherapy, diathermy. Since "one or more sessions" is already in the description, a modifier is not needed. Also, if Evaluation and Management services are performed by the same physician in more than one location, many payers will combine the two services into one code for reporting. For example, when an office visit results in an admission to the hospital on the same date, both codes should not be reported unless they are significantly and separately identifiable from each other.

3. Modifiers should be used to increase or reduce a service only when no other code describes the extent of the procedure. When lymph nodes are removed in addition to a mastectomy for a breast malignancy, a more comprehensive code such as 19240 (Mastectomy, modified radical, including axillary lymph nodes. . .) should be used instead of mastectomy codes 19180 or 19182 with a modifier. The modifier for reduced services (-52) is not appropriate for a service where only the fee is reduced or a code exists that specifically describes the circumstances.

4. Bilateral modifiers are not reported when the CPT code description includes the word "bilateral" or the phrase "unilateral or bilateral." For example, code 55450 (Ligation, percutaneous of vas deferens, unilateral or bilateral) would never have modifier -50 appended since the code already indicates the procedure may be bilateral.

REQUIRED REPORTING FORMATS AND REIMBURSEMENT IMPACT

The CPT manual allows modifiers to be reported two different ways, but third party payers may restrict reporting options to accommodate their information system requirements. The two-digit modifier may be placed in field 24-D of the HCFA 1500 for physician reporting. Modifiers may be listed adjacent to the CPT code and separated by a hyphen for narrative reporting purposes. For example: Bilateral myringotomy with tube placement 69436-50. A separate code using 09950 is also permissible, according to CPT. The same procedure as above would be reported 69436 on one line with 09950 on the next line. Individual payers may not recognize CPT modifiers at all or may have their own rules for modifier reporting at variance with CPT guidelines. For example, for a number of years CPT allowed reporting of bilateral procedures such as the myringotomy with tubes using either a one-line (69436-50) or a two-line method (69436 for the first ear and 69436-50 for the second, bilateral procedure). For many health plans, the first code would be reimbursed at 100 percent of the allowed fee schedule amount and the second code would be reduced by 50 percent to compensate for the overlapping preoperative and postoperative services. The September, 1997, *CPT Assistant* (Volume 7, Issue 9, p. 4) clarified this reporting rule and stated "The intent of CPT is that a single-line method be used (i.e., 12345-50)." Despite this intent, some insurance plans require a two-line method of reporting, which creates data quality concerns in some provider organizations. Reimbursement is affected by certain modifiers that multiply the allowed amounts or reduce the allowed amounts by defined percentages. Other modifiers do not affect payments directly, but assist in getting the claim paid by explaining certain payment conditions that determine whether the service is reimbursed or denied.

In a study conducted by the AMA and reported in the September, 1997, *CPT Assistant,* various rates of modifier acceptance by payers were reported, with the highest acceptance rate attributed to Medicare (86 percent) and the lowest to Medicaid (45 percent) claim processors ("Readers Respond to Faxback Survey on Modifiers," *CPT Assistant*, Volume 7, Issue 9, pp. 6-7).

HCFA allows reporting of up to four two-digit modifiers on the HCFA 1500, but a maximum of two two-digit modifiers for hospital reporting on the UB-92 (HCFA 1450 form). CPT has a mechanism to report multiple modifiers by first reporting 09999 or appending modifier -99 to the CPT code. Modifier -99 is not necessary if the third party payer's computer system accepts multiple modifiers on the same line of the HCFA form. If the system does not allow reporting this way, modifier -99 is appended to the basic service and all applicable additional modifiers are added in the appropriate location on the form. HCFA does not allow the multiple modifier code for hospital modifier reporting.

Physician Use of CPT Modifiers

The most prevalent use of CPT modifiers is for the reporting of physician services. Facility services are, by nature, not as likely to require modification from the code description since facility services reimbursement is less likely to be affected by special circumstances. Modifiers for professional services define unusual cases, mandated services, times when a decision for surgery is made, or services that are separate from others and deserve consideration for payment.

ASC Use of CPT Modifiers

Ambulatory Surgery Centers use selected modifiers similar to hospital outpatient requirements for HCFA reporting. In the past, only HCPCS modifiers applied for reporting facility services in ASC locations not affiliated with a hospital.

Hospital Use of CPT Modifiers

Hospitals report only a subset of CPT modifiers. Reporting by hospitals and ASCs was implemented in 1998 preceding introduction of the APC (Ambulatory Payment Classification) system for HCFA reimbursement of Medicare beneficiaries receiving outpatient facility services. The following CPT modifiers were introduced for hospital and/or ASC reporting:

- -50 Bilateral Procedures
- -52 Reduced Procedures
- -53 Discontinued Procedures (Revised to modifiers -73 and -74 in 1999)
- -59 Distinct/Separate Procedures
- -76 Repeat Procedures, Same Physician
- -77 Repeat Procedures, Different Physician

In 1999, modifier -73 discontinued outpatient hospital/ASC procedure before anesthesia, and -74 discontinued outpatient hospital/ASC procedure after anesthesia. A number of HCPCS Level II modifiers are also reportable to HCFA for Medicare patients. Acceptance of either the CPT or HCPCS modifiers for other payers is not known at the time of this writing. Refer to Appendix A for currently available modifiers.

According to the proposed rules for APC-based prospective payment, the direct impact of modifiers results in the use of the first three procedures by indicating full allowance (100 percent) or half allowance (50 percent) of allowed benefits will be paid for the APC group generated by the CPT code(s) involved. The other modifiers do not have a direct monetary impact, but may facilitate claim payment by avoiding medical review processes in situations where reimbursement is justified by medical necessity of the separate or repeated procedure during the same operative session or on the same date of service.

In July, 1998, Medicare implemented the use of hospital-specific modifiers. Two of these modifiers— -52 and -53—had HCFA descriptions that were at variance with the CPT definition. The 1999 version of CPT makes it easy to distinguish hospital-reported modifiers by creating a special section entitled: "Modifiers Approved for Ambulatory Surgery Center (ASC) Hospital Outpatient Use." Two new modifiers have been created so that the CPT definitions can remain constant. Modifiers -73 and -74 have been added to CPT with the HCFA definitions included.

It should be noted that the use of five digits to communicate modifiers is not permitted for HCFA patients. The directive requires use of the two-digit modifiers appended to the CPT codes on the UB-92.

HCPCS Modifiers Also Appear

For the first time in CPT history, HCPCS modifiers have been added to Appendix A in a special Hospital section. This is a list of the approved national modifiers required by HCFA for reporting after July 1, 1998. This is not a complete list, since only hospital modifiers are included rather than the full set used by other types of health care providers.

TABLE 8.1   Selected Modifiers with Coding and Reimbursement Tips

Modifier	Description	Applicable CPT Range	Reimbursement or Billing Tips	Example
-21	Prolonged Evaluation and Management Services	May only be listed with the highest level of E/M service.	Most payers consider this modifier to be informational only and do not provide additional payment when it is reported. Prolonged E/M service codes (99354-99359) replace use of this modifier in most cases. The AMA indicates that -21 is only used when physician-patient contact is continuous, while prolonged service codes may be used when the contact is either continuous or intermittent. HCFA does not allow extra payment for this modifier. Use only with the highest level of E/M code for the service reported. Examples: 99205, 99215, 99220, 99223, 99245, 99255, etc. This modifier is not reported by hospitals.	An elderly patient is visited by her internist in the skilled care unit to evaluate diabetic ulcers and cellulitis of the feet. A comprehensive detailed interval history is taken, a comprehensive physician examination is performed, and medical decision making of moderate complexity is documented in the record. Following the patient exam, the physician spends an additional 30 minutes with the patient and/or family discussing treatment options and future care plans for a total of 55 minutes. Since this service is greater than the CPT code 99313 (Subsequent nursing facility care), modifier -21 could be appended to the code to indicate a prolonged service.
-22	Unusual Procedural Services	Attached to a code when services(s) provided is greater than that usually required for a listed procedure.	Used to alert payers to unusual circumstances or complications encountered during a procedure. Use of this modifier invites individual consideration and manual review. Payers watch use of this modifier very carefully since it has been widely abused. These words in an operative report help document unusual circumstances: "increased risk," "difficult," "extended," "complications," "prolonged," "severe respiratory distress," "hemorrhage," "blood loss over 600 cc," "unusual findings," or "unusual contamination controls." HCFA contends that the slight extension of a procedure does not warrant the -22 modifier. The circumstance must involve significant increase in physician work.	Use modifier -22 when: • complications cannot be identified by a separate code and there is a significant increase in physician work; • the procedure is lengthy and unusual; or • work and effort are increased by approximately 30-50 percent of what would normally be required due to unusual circumstances. Send a cover letter and report with the claim documenting unusual circumstances; do not use generalizations, e.g., "Surgery took an extra 90 minutes," "This was a difficult surgery," or "The patient was very sick." BE SPECIFIC! (For example: it is helpful to state that the procedure took 3 hours and normally only takes 1 hour. Show the payer how the work was increased. Instead of transmitting electronically, use a "paper claim" with attached documentation for consideration.) HCFA may increase reimbursement if sufficient documentation is submitted. Use modifier -22 on procedure codes with a global fee period when unusual circumstances warrant consideration of payment in excess of fee schedule allowances due to complications. This modifier is not reported by hospitals.

Modifier	Description	Applicable CPT Range	Reimbursement or Billing Tips	Example
-23	Unusual Anesthesia	Only reportable with anesthesia codes.	Not reported by surgeons. Anesthesiologists or anesthetists only may report this modifier. Do not use for local anesthesia. Documentation should be submitted with the claim for service. This modifier is not reported by hospitals. Use this modifier when a procedure usually requires no anesthetic or local anesthesia, but in this situation requires general anesthesia.	A six-year-old child is examined in the ER with a foreign body in the ear. Because the child is not cooperative, a general anesthetic is required to allow the ER physician to remove the object.
-24	Unrelated E/M Service by the Same Physician During a Postoperative Period	Attach to an E/M service provided during a postoperative period.	Do not attach to a CPT surgical procedure code. Must be linked with a diagnosis code that indicates the service is unrelated to the surgery. HCFA authorizes payments for in-patient services with modifier -24 for the following special circumstances: • Immunotherapy furnished by the transplant surgeon; • Critical care for a burn or trauma patient, although documentation must accompany the claim; or • When diagnosis coding supports the claim that the E/M service is unrelated to the surgery. If the original surgeon readmits the patient during the postoperative global period, he or she attaches modifier -24 to the E/M service and documents that the patient's condition is unrelated to the surgery. If a different physician is admitting the patient, modifier -24 is not used. This modifier should not be used to obtain reimbursement in the postoperative period for cataract patients when a comprehensive eye examination has preceded the decision for the patient to have both eyes operated on. After the first eye is completed, the opthalmologist has the patient return postoperatively and makes plans to perform the cataract surgery on the other eye. Unless there is a significant change in diagnosis warranting another comprehensive examination, reporting of an Evaluation and Management code with this modifier is not appropriate, according to some Medicare carrier policies. Because CPT does not define the number of days in a postoperative period, you must determine the payer's	A patient at the 75th postoperative day following a prostatectomy is admitted for sharp abdominal pains, primarily in the right flank. Further workup revealed a calculus in the ureter. No surgery is recommended, but continued observation and pain control is warranted, so the patient is admitted to observation status at the hospital. The physician will report the observation code (99218-99220) with modifier -24 and the diagnosis code for the calculus linked with it to avoid denials from the payer for routine follow-up services.

Modifier	Description	Applicable CPT Range	Reimbursement or Billing Tips	Example
			definition before coding the case. Subsequent hospital care (99231-99233, 99291-99292) by the surgeon during the same hospitalization as the surgery is considered related to the surgery. Separate payment for such a visit is not allowed even when billed with the -24 modifier unless one of the following conditions listed above applies to the case.	A patient comes to the office for a scheduled removal of a benign cyst excision on the arm. Following the procedure, he asks the physician to examine his back which he strained three weeks ago and has caused him to lose sleep due to severe pain. The physician performs an expanded problem focused history and examination for these complaints and documents medical decision making at the low level. Code 99213-25 may be reported in addition to code 11400 for the cyst excision. Two different diagnosis codes will be reported, with the back strain code linked to the office visit code on the HCFA 1500 form.
			This modifier is not reported by hospitals.	
-25	Significant, Separately Identifiable E/M Service by the Same Physician on the Same Day of the Procedure or Other Service	E/M Codes only	The language for this modifier was revised in 1995 CPT with "or other service" added. This allows the reporting of a problem or abnormality picked up during a preventative medicine visit that is significant enough to require additional work to perform the key components of a problem or E/M service. Report this "significant and separately identifiable E/M service" with -25. (Do not report additional E/M service if a problem is identified but nothing is done about it).	A parent schedules an appointment for a well-child physical. During the encounter, which includes a history and physical exam relevant to the child's age, the parent mentions that the child complains consistently about leg pain and cramping. Further evaluation is conducted to respond to this symptom, including a detailed H&P and medical decision making of moderate level due to the number of possible diagnoses and management options and the tests ordered to rule out certain conditions. Code 99392 is assigned for the well-child check up and code 99214-25 is reported for the E/M service unrelated to the routine care. Third party payer rules may vary
			Modifier -25 may be attached to an E/M service code representing a significant, separately identifiable service performed on the same day as routine foot care. The visit must be medically necessary for another problem. The routine care is the patient's responsibility, according to Medicare rules. The E/M service should be unrelated to the other procedure or service that is provided.	concerning this reporting, as some plans would expect one service or the other to be allowed, rather than both. Preventive care often has different payment requirements for copayments and deductibles. Some plans would not allow charging the full fee for both services, and would expect the charge to be reduced
			Upfront documentation is not required; however, distinguishing diagnosis codes should be provided when available. HCFA does not allow additional reimbursement for this modifier, but use of it may prevent denial of office visit codes on the same date as a procedure when separate work is done. There is a difference between the AMA CPT definition and Medicare rules for use of this modifier. Medicare guidelines instruct codes to use -25 if a decision for surgery is made on the same day as a minor procedure. This modifier may be appended to critical care codes 99291-99292 to indicate services provided during a global period to a seriously injured or burned patient.	

Modifier	Description	Applicable CPT Range	Reimbursement or Billing Tips	Example
		E/M Codes only	The diagnosis code linked to the services is important in avoiding denial for bundled services. When this modifier is used, the key elements of history, examination, and medical decision making should be clearly documented for the service reported separately. Application of initial casts and strapping (CPT codes 29075 and 29125) by an emergency department physician can be separately reported in certain circumstances. When the ER physician is not providing the entire global care or intraoperative service of fracture care but applies the cast/strapping, then the E/M service can be reported using modifier -25. This modifier is not used for hospital reporting yet, although it was mentioned in the proposed regulations for APCs. The application mentioned says that "in cases where a surgical procedure or service is performed as the immediate result of an outpatient visit (such as removal of skin lesions following a visit to a dermatology clinic) or from an emergency department visit, the visit would be reported with modifier -25." This indicates to Medicare that a separately identifiable E/M service was furnished that merits an APC payment over and above the payment for surgery.	due to overlap in the preventive care and problem-oriented care history and physical examination work. A patient presents to the ER with a serious hand and finger laceration requiring immediate operative intervention. Before going to surgery, initial evaluation and stabilization took place in the emergency department. Later in the day, an orthopedic hand specialist was available and the patient received outpatient surgery before being dismissed on the same date. Modifier -25, if accepted for hospital use, could be used in this situation to prevent denial of the ER service with a surgical service on the same date.
-26	Professional Component	Modifier -26 is used when it is necessary to separate the professional component from the technical component for a given service.	A re-read of results of another physician's interpretation should not be reported this way. This is a common modifier for radiologists, cardiologists, and other specialty physicians who perform diagnostic workups on someone else's equipment, using someone else's staff, such as a hospital or free-standing diagnostic center. Do not assign this modifier to codes that already describe interpretation and reporting as separate from the technical portion of the service. To use this modifier and receive reimbursement for professional services, a signed written report must be prepared that includes findings, relevant clinical issues, and comparative data, as appropriate. A review of the procedure findings with a written report for confirmation does not meet the requirements for reporting a code with this modifier.	A complex cystometrogram is performed by a urologist in the hospital outpatient radiology department. Code 51726-26 is reported since the urologist operated the hospital equipment and interpreted the results but did not provide the technical component of the service. The hospital would report the same code for the technical component using 51726-TC for a Medicare patient. Hospitals cannot report this modifier, since it would be inappropriate for facility services.

Modifier	Description	Applicable CPT Range	Reimbursement or Billing Tips	Example
			These services and/or notations would be considered by third party payers to be included in E/M services reported on that date of service.	
-32	Mandated Service	N/A	Peer review organizations' (PROs) requests may be identified by adding this modifier to consultation services or related procedures that are required to meet agency needs. A common use of this modifier is for workers compensation cases when the carrier wants the patient to seek the opinion of a different doctor before going ahead with surgery or other expensive treatments. This is not a modifier used for second opinion requests from the patient or his or her family. Waiver of copayments and deductibles is often granted when this modifier is used; otherwise there is no effect on payment amounts. Hospitals may not report this modifier.	A known child molester was ordered to undergo court-ordered castration. Code 54520-32 is reported for the physician services since the service is mandated. A 40-year-old female patient desires a hysterectomy. Her insurance plan requires a second opinion before they will certify the procedure and pay for it. Code 99243-32 is submitted for the office consultation which included a detailed history, a detailed physical exam, and medical decision making of low complexity.
-47	Anesthesia by Surgeon	This modifier is added when the anesthesia is administered by the operating physician.	HCFA does not provide additional payment for this service. Other payer policies may vary. This code should not be reported unless payment rules allow separate reimbursement or there is a particular need to track the incidence of this service. Use of this modifier denotes regional or general anesthesia, since local anesthesia is by CPT definition included in a surgery. This modifier is only applied to surgery codes, not anesthesia codes. This modifier is not reported by hospitals.	A gastroenterologist administers IV Versed in order to perform an upper GI endoscopy for removal of an esophageal polyp with a snare. The CPT code is listed twice; once for the procedure 43217, and then with the modifier for the anesthesia administration, 43217-47. This is only for the reporting for the physician services. When reporting hospital services the code is listed only once.
-50	Bilateral Service	This modifier is used by physicians and by hospitals for reporting procedures performed on both sides of the body where the code description is not specific to laterality.	Payment by HCFA is 150 percent for procedures that allow this modifier. HCFA considers many ophthalmological procedures (92002-92499) to be bilateral; if the procedure is performed on only one eye, then modifier -52 (reduced services) should be used for physician reporting. For hospital reporting, see the HCFA requirements for	Bilateral myringotomy 69436-50.

Modifier	Description	Applicable CPT Range	Reimbursement or Billing Tips	Example
			modifier -52 that are slightly different than CPT modifier requirements.	
			There are times when surgery is performed on both sides of the body that may appear to be bilateral, but in truth, can be considered multiple procedures. One example is surgery involving the turbinates (they are also called conchas). There are six turbinates, three on each side: two superior, two middle, and two inferior. If a surgeon removes both superior turbinates, for example, this is considered bilateral, and modifier -50 would be used. However, if one superior and one middle and/or inferior turbinates are removed from the other side, these would be considered multiple procedures, with one billing 100 percent of the fee, and each additional billed with -51. If there were two turbinates in opposite positions, superior, middle or inferior, this would be bilateral (-50), and any other additional removal would use -51. The operative notes should clearly state the number and position of each turbinate removed for accurate billing.	
			Medicare has a listing of procedure codes in the Medicare Physicians' Fee Data Base (MPFDB). An indicator of "1" in this list means that 150 percent of the fee schedule amount will be paid. An indicator of "2" means that the payment adjustment will not apply since the RVUs are already based on the procedure being performed on both sides. One hundred percent of the single code fee amounts is all that will be reimbursed. An indicator of "3" means that the usual payment adjustment for bilateral procedures does not apply to a specific code. An indicator of "9" means that the bilateral concept does not apply to this code. These indicators apply to physician reporting of services only. Use of modifier -50 would not be appropriate when reporting lesion removal on the right arm and the left arm, even if the lesions were identical in size and pathology. The skin is considered one body organ in CPT.	
			Use modifier -50 only when the exact same procedure is reported for each site.	

Modifier	Description	Applicable CPT Range	Reimbursement or Billing Tips	Example
			Lacrimal punctal plugs are coded 68761 which includes closure of a single punctum. If this procedure is performed on both eyes, modifier -50 is appropriate. CPT guidelines and HCFA regulations state that only one CPT code is used to report a bilateral procedure on one line of a HCFA 1500. HCFA requests a unit of "1" be used in the units field for a bilateral procedure reported on one line with modifier -50 appended. Other commercial payers may have different requirements, such as listing the code twice with the -50 modifier only on the second code. Some ask for placement of a "2" in the "units" field on the HCFA. Payer requirements must be verified before reporting.	
-51	Multiple Procedures	N/A	Use this modifier to denote more than one medical/surgical procedure being performed by the same physician on the same day at the same operative session. The major procedure is listed first and is reimbursed in full. Secondary or lesser procedures may be listed next with modifier -51.	Tonsillectomy and adenoidectomy and myringtomy at the same operative session. Modifier -51 is appended to the lesser value procedure.
			Appendix F in CPT lists procedures that are exempt from use of modifier -51.	
			HCFA pays 100 percent for the first procedure and 50 percent for the second through fifth procedures for physician services. More than one hospital service is not reported by modifier use. Any other multiple procedures will be paid after carrier review. Special rules apply for billing dermatology and endoscopy procedures. Attachment of this modifier to an anesthesiology procedure does not affect payment. When billing, do not reduce the payment; allow the payer to do so. This modifier is not reported by hospitals.	
-52	Reduced Services	This modifier is used by physicians and is available for reporting by hospitals in selected circumstances.	Use to denote a partially reduced or eliminated procedure or service due to physician's election or the patient's emotional status.	Procedures that are normally performed bilaterally but are only performed on one side. Procedure not completed due to patient's condition.
				Use of ICD-9-CM code will identify reason for reduction of service. See code range in category V64.X

Modifier	Description	Applicable CPT Range	Reimbursement or Billing Tips	Example
			Report the appropriate ICD-9-CM code V64.1, V64.2, or V64.3 to indicate that the procedure was not carried out as planned. This modifier applies to procedures in the physician's office or to procedures performed in an ASC or Out-patient Radiology Departments.	(Persons encountering health services for specific procedures, not carried out). HCFA considers exams as global procedures and attachment of this modifier will not affect payment; however, if this modifier is attached to aborted procedures, reduction in payment may occur, so documentation should be submitted.
-53	Discontinued Procedure		This modifier is used for physician service reporting. Hospitals use modifier -74 for discontinued or terminated procedures. Used for reporting extenuating circumstances or those that threaten the well-being of the patient when the physician elects to terminate a surgical or diagnostic procedure.	In an ENT clinic, a patient was undergoing a nasal endoscopy, when the endoscope malfunctioned before the procedure was completed. Modifier -53 is appended to code 31231.
-54	Surgical Care Only	N/A	This modifier indicates that more than one physician is involved in a patient's surgical care and this physician is the one performing the operative services. Use when one physician provides surgical services and another provides preoperative and/or postoperative care. The medical record should contain a written agreement for transfer of care. It is generally understood that modifier -54 includes the preoperative care that a surgeon renders the day before surgery as well as the surgical services. HCFA indicates that payment will be limited to the preoperative and intraoperative services only. This modifier is not reported by hospitals.	An orthopedic surgeon that only provides OR care and not other services.

Modifier	Description	Applicable CPT Range	Reimbursement or Billing Tips	Example
-55	Postoperative Management Only	N/A	This modifier indicates that multiple physicians are involved in the patient's surgical care and this physician is only managing postoperative services. Use when one physician provides only the postoperative care and deserves the postoperative percentage of the global service. Do not attach this modifier to an E/M service code; it is only attached to the surgical or medical procedure code (include the date the surgery was performed). May only be billed after the first postoperative visit has been performed. HCFA indicates that payment is limited to the amount allotted for postoperative services only.	Optometrists may use this modifier when postoperative cataract care is provided and care is transferred to them. This modifier is not reported by hospitals.
-56	Preoperative Management Only	Attach this modifier to the surgical or medical procedure code.	Use of this modifier indicates that other physicians were responsible for the intraoperative and postoperative care of the patient. This modifier is rarely used since it is generally understood that the operating physician includes preoperative management in conjunction with the surgery by many health plans. Do not use this modifier for Medicare claims, since payment for this component is included in the allowed amount for the surgery. This modifier is not reported by hospitals.	A surgeon prepares patient for surgery but becomes ill and cannot perform the procedure. Preoperative services may be billed with modifier -56.
-57	Decision for Surgery	Identifies an E/M service that resulted in the decision for surgery during the preoperative global period (the day before or day of surgery). Attach this modifier to an E/M service code, not the procedure code.	HCFA expects this modifier to be used when the surgery has a 90-day postoperative period. Use of this modifier does not affect payment, but may prevent denial of services as included in the global fee. This modifier is used only in cases in which a decision for surgery was made during the preoperative period of a surgical procedure with a 90-day global period for Medicare reporting. It should not be used with visits furnished during the global period of minor procedures (0 or 10 day global). HCFA instructs providers to use modifier -25 for this purpose when documentation is available that	Consultation by orthopedic surgeon before fracture reduction.

Modifier	Description	Applicable CPT Range	Reimbursement or Billing Tips	Example
			substantiates significant, separately identifiable services. This modifier is not reported by hospitals.	
-58	Staged or Related Procedure or Service by the Same Physician During the Postoperative Period	Use this modifier when a procedure is performed during the postoperative period and was planned prospectively at the time of the original procedure, is more extensive than the original procedure, or is used for therapy following a diagnostic surgical procedure which has a global period.	HCFA has clarified that surgical procedures which contain the language "one or more sessions," e.g., codes 67141-67228, should not be modified with -58. Also do not use this modifier on Mohs' micrographic surgery (17304-17310). HCFA has indicated that use of this modifier does not affect payment. Hospitals may not report this modifier.	Sternal debridement (21627) is performed to remove infected tissue. At the time of the procedure, it is noted that a muscle flap repair will be required in several days to close the defect. Code 15734-58 is reported since the procedure was planned at the time of first procedure.
-59	Distinct Procedural Service		This modifier may be used by both hospitals and physicians. Its purpose is to identify a procedure or service distinct or independent of other services performed at the same time or on the same date.

If there is any other modifier that is more descriptive than this one it should be used rather than modifier -59. When a procedure in CPT is designated as a "separate procedure" this modifier can be used to explain that in this circumstance, the procedure was carried out independently, or distinct from another service that it normally would be considered integral to. The modifier indicates that it is appropriate to report the procedure in addition to the more comprehensive code because it is distinct from the other procedure. The CPT codes for use with modifier -59 are 00100-01999, 10040-69979, 70010-79999, 80049-89399, and 90700-99199, unless the payer in question limits modifier reporting.

Modifier -59 is not used on E/M codes for physician services. It is appropriately used when a billing combination of codes exists which would normally not occur together. The modifier indicates that the ordinarily bundled code represents a service done at a different time, performed on a different site, or in a separate session on the same date. | |

Modifier	Description	Applicable CPT Range	Reimbursement or Billing Tips	Example
			Medicare uses the National Correct Coding Initiative to determine bundled services. Use of this modifier causes these edits to be bypassed so it is critical that documentation be present that validates the separate reporting of bundled services for payment. Hospitals use this modifier to allow additional payment for services that are usually bundled into the more comprehensive code.	
			In the APC system, it is expected that the NCCI bundling edits will be utilized to control unbundling by the hospital for facility services.	
-62	Two Surgeons	Surgery Codes	This modifier is used only when the skills of two surgeons are required to accomplish a single procedure. Cosurgeries are usually performed by physicians of different specialties on the same case. When the services are different and result in separate CPT codes, this modifier is not used.	
			Surgeons must have equal participation in the procedure in question. This modifier is not intended for a surgeon–assistant surgeon relationship. Dates of service must match for both claims for services when separate billing is performed for services. Use of this modifier is limited to surgical services only.	
			Documentation is often required to substantiate the need for two surgeons.	
			For Medicare cases, each surgeon receives 62.5 percent of the allowed amount for the CPT code in question when this modifier is used. This modifier is not reported by hospitals.	
-66	Surgical Team	This modifier is restricted to reporting of highly complex procedures that require a special team of physicians.	The modifier is appended to the CPT code(s) reported by each member of the team. Individual health plans may have specific reimbursement guidelines for team surgery that apply. For Medicare, the carrier determines what the payment will be for selected surgeries where a surgical team is required.	

Modifier	Description	Applicable CPT Range	Reimbursement or Billing Tips	Example
-73	Discontinued Out-Patient Hospital/Ambulatory Surgery Center (ASC) Procedure Prior to the Administration of Anesthesia	ASC or Hospital Services only	Due to extenuating circumstances, or those that threaten the well-being of the patient, the physician may cancel a surgical or diagnostic procedure subsequent to the patient's surgical preparation (including sedation, when provided, and being taken to the room where the procedure is to be performed), but prior to the administration of anesthesia (local, regional block(s) or general). Under these circumstances, the intended service that is prepared for but cancelled can be reported by the usual procedure number and the addition of modifier -73 or by the use of the separate five-digit modifier 09973. Note: The elective cancellation of a service prior to the administration of anesthesia and/or surgical preparation of the patient should not be reported. For physician reporting of a discontinued procedure see modifier -53.	A hospital out-patient surgery is planned for a patient to receive phacoemulsification of left eye cataract with lens replacement. Before the retrobulbar block was administered, the patient became short of breath and her heart rate increased. The procedure was cancelled pending further workup of symptoms. Code 66984-73 is assigned.
-74	Discontinued Out-Patient Hospital/Ambulatory Surgery Center (ASC) Procedure After the Administration of Anesthesia	ASC or Hospital Services only	Due to extenuating circumstances, or those that threaten the well-being of the patient, the physician may terminate a surgical or diagnostic procedure after the administration of anesthesia (local, regional block(s) or general) or after the procedure was started (incision made, intubation started, scope inserted, etc.). Under these circumstances, the intended service that is started but terminated can be reported by the usual procedure number and the addition of modifier -74 or by the use of the separate five-digit modifier 09974. Note: The elective cancellation of a service prior to the administration of anesthesia and/or surgical preparation of the patient should not be reported. For physician reporting of a discontinued procedure see modifier -53.	A hospital out-patient surgery is planned for a patient to receive phacoemulsification of left eye cataract. *After* the retrobulbar block was administered the patient became short of breath *and* her heart rate increased. The procedure was cancelled pending further workup of symptoms. Code 66984-74 is reported.
-76	Repeat Procedure by Same Physician	This modifier is used by physicians and hospitals to indicate that a procedure had to be repeated.	This helps to prevent denials for duplicate services, when the health plan is unaware that more than one service is being reported, often on the same date. Use to report a repeat procedure by the same physician performed subsequent (usually the same day) to the original procedure. HCFA has indicated that this modifier does not affect payment and is for informational purposes only.	Used to report repeat laboratory procedures, e.g., repeat blood sugars that are medically necessary on the same date. The modifier is used to prevent claim denial for duplicate billing, which is part of the edits in place by the carrier for inappropriate billing.

Modifier	Description	Applicable CPT Range	Reimbursement or Billing Tips	Example
			Hospitals may report this service. The HCFA mandate states that "a procedure or service was repeated in a separate operative session on the same day." Hospitals are to report the first procedure and then list it again with the modifier appended to report the subsequent procedure. The actual number of times the procedure was repeated is to be added in the units field of the UB-92. For ASC-covered procedures the units field is not used; instead, the code is listed as many times as the procedure was repeated with the modifier appended to the second and each subsequent procedure code.	
-77	Repeat Procedure by Another Physician	Surgery/Radiology Codes	Identical to modifier -76 except that the physician is different from the one who performed the original service. HCFA indicates that use of this modifier does not affect payment. Hospitals may report this service. The HCFA mandate states that "a procedure or service was repeated in a separate operative session on the same day." Hospitals are to report the first procedure and then list it again with the modifier appended to report the subsequent procedure. The actual number of times the procedure was repeated is to be added in the units field. For ASC-covered procedures, the units field is not used. The code is listed once for the first procedure and then the repeated procedures are reported, each one with modifier -77 appended.	A primary care physician performs a chest X-ray in his office and observes a suspicious mass. He sends the patient to a pulmonologist who, on the same day, repeats the chest X-ray. The pulmonologist would submit his claim with modifier -77 and documentation.
-78	Return to the Operating Room for a Related Procedure During the Postoperative Period	Surgery Codes	"Operating room" is defined by HCFA as a place of service specifically equipped and staffed for the sole purpose of performing procedures. This includes cardiac catheterization suites, laser suites, and endoscopy suites. It does not include a patient room, a minor treatment room, a recovery room, or an intensive care unit. Use this modifier to report the treatment of a problem that requires a return to the operating room and is related to the original procedure, e.g., medical, surgical, or mechanical complications.	A patient who had a total knee replacement performed 1/26/99 requires a return to surgery on 2/2/99 for revision of one component. Code 27486-78 is reported.

Modifier	Description	Applicable CPT Range	Reimbursement or Billing Tips	Example
			HCFA allows 50 percent of the intraoperative amount and recognizes this modifier when attached to procedures with a 10- or 90-day global period. A new postoperative period does not begin with the use of modifier -78. HCFA allows full payment for complications treated by another physician if expertise beyond that of the first surgeon is necessary to treat the complication. In this case, no modifier is needed and only the allowance for the intraoperative period will be allowed. This modifier is not reported by hospitals.	
-79	Unrelated Procedure or Service by the Same Physician During the Postoperative Period	N/A	This modifier is similar to modifier -78 except that the return to the operating room is for an unrelated procedure and this modifier specifies that the physician is the same one who performed the original surgery. Indicate that the procedure is unrelated by using a correct diagnosis code. With -79, a new postoperative period begins and payment should be the full amount. This modifier should not be used to denote a return to the operating room for complications due to the original surgery. HCFA has indicated that use of this modifier does not affect the payment amount. Hospitals may not report this modifier.	A patient received an open treatment of a femoral fracture on Feb. 1, 1999. On Feb. 14 he slipped while on crutches and fractured the other leg, requiring a return trip to the OR for percutaneous skeletal fixation. Code 27509-79 is reported for the second procedure. HCPCS modifiers for RT (right) or LT (left) may also assist in reporting.
-80	Assistant Surgeon	Surgery Codes	This modifier may be added to the surgical code to indicate that the reporting physician is assisting at surgery. Medicare and many insurance plans do not allow payment for surgical assist services by non-licensed physicians or nonphysicians. Even Certified Surgical Assistants are not approved for Medicare benefits. Physician Assistants may qualify for some reimbursement by following specific Medicare rules for reporting with HCPCS modifiers. Medicare has a list of surgical codes where an assistant is approved for reimbursement. It is based on national utilization of assistants. When the statistic drops below	Assistant at C-Section delivery (no prenatal or postnatal care). Code 59514-80 is reported.

Modifier	Description	Applicable CPT Range	Reimbursement or Billing Tips	Example
			5 percent, no additional reimbursement is allowed without documentation of medical necessity.	
			Medicare reimbursement is 16 percent of the global amount approved for surgery in 1998.	
			This modifier is restricted to surgical code ranges 10040-69979 or radiology procedures that may be interventional in nature and require an assistant. It would be inappropriate for a hospital to report this modifier.	
-81	Assistant Minimum Surgeon	Surgery Codes	This modifier is occasionally used to report the assistance of another surgeon for a relatively short period of time during the procedure.	Any surgical procedure where a brief assistance is rendered. This is not the same as modifier -80 for a full assist.
			This modifier rarely would be reimbursed by Medicare or other payers. It would be inappropriate for a hospital to report this modifier.	
-82	Assistant Surgeon (Qualified Resident Not Available)	Surgery Codes	This modifier is often used in medical centers, where teaching surgeons utilize residents to assist at surgery. In a teaching hospital Medicare assumes that a qualified resident is not available unless a certification is on file for each claim. This certification has prescribed language that must be followed.	Any surgery where conditions are met.
			This modifier is only used on the surgical code ranges 10040-69979, as appropriate. If it is used consistently at a teaching hospital, it would invite an audit by Medicare or other insurance plans. It would be inappropriate for a hospital to report this modifier.	
-90	Reference Laboratory	In General Lab Procedures	This modifier is added to the usual procedure code for laboratory procedures performed by a party other than the treating or reporting physician.	CBC sent to reference lab by physician office. 85025-90
			Add to lab tests when billing and reporting for the test is desired, or when the test has been purchased from an outside reference lab.	

Modifier	Description	Applicable CPT Range	Reimbursement or Billing Tips	Example
			Medicare does not allow billing for laboratory tests if a physician's office does not perform it. The entity providing the test is the one that must bill for it unless the service is provided under "acceptable arrangements" defined by HCFA.	
			This modifier is most appropriate with the 80049-89399 range of codes, but may also be used with surgical, radiology, and medical procedure codes when the circumstances apply. Hospitals may not report this modifier.	
-99	Multiple Modifiers	Attach to a service/procedure code when two or more modifiers are necessary to describe the service performed.	This modifier is rarely used; payers have different instructions regarding where to list additional modifiers. Hospitals may not report this modifier. HCFA mandates allow only two modifiers per code for hospital reporting.	Use on the rare occasion of reporting two or more modifiers for the same code.

100

Review Exercises Using Modifiers

1. If modifier -50 is attached to code 69436, which results in an APC 313 reimbursement of $383.95, and the payer using the APC system reduces payment for multiple procedure APC groups to 50 percent, what will the expected payment be for the code with the modifier?
   a. $767.90
   b. $575.93
   c. $191.98
   d. $383.95

2. What modifier is used when a physician's office does not own any lab equipment, yet chooses to bill for lab services they purchase from a supplier?
   a. Modifier -59 Separate procedure
   b. Modifier -22 Unusual services
   c. Modifier -52 Reduced services
   d. Modifier -90 Reference (outside) laboratory

3. What code and modifier(s) would be used by a podiatrist when he or she performs bunion correction with sesamoidectomy and exostectomy, both feet?
   a. 28288-52
   b. 28299-51
   c. 28296-50
   d. 28290-50

4. A series of chest X-rays is taken for a patient with severe cardiomyopathy to monitor pleural effusion. Which modifier might the interpreting radiologist want to include on the second reading on the first day of hospitalization?
   a. -58 Staged procedure
   b. -76 Repeat procedure, same physician
   c. -59 Distinct procedure
   d. No modifier is necessary.

5. An ophthalmologist and an optometrist work together in the same office but are not partners and have separate provider contracts. After a patient has cataract surgery, the optometrist provides the required follow-up care. What modifier is used on the codes reported for his services?
   a. -55 Postoperative management only
   b. -56 Preoperative management only
   c. -22 Unusual procedure
   d. -52 Reduced service

Appendix

Comprehensive Coding Review Exercises

This appendix contains review exercises to aid in preparation for a coding certification examination or for assessment of basic CPT guidelines and application of coding principles.

1. In the 1999 edition of CPT, revisions to the appendices were made. Which one of these represented a significant change from older versions of CPT?
   a. Appendix A had selected modifiers deleted, but none added.
   b. Appendix B was unusually brief.
   c. Appendix E and F were added for "add-on codes" and "exempt from modifier -51" codes.
   d. Appendix C was revised to include complete descriptions.

2. Which of the following statements is true?
   a. HCPCS codes are interchangeable with CPT codes.
   b. Hospital use of CPT requires a different set of guidelines.
   c. CPT comprises Level I of HCPCS and is administered by the AMA.
   d. When a procedure has a CPT code, Medicare coverage is assured.

3. In the Integumentary section of CPT, excision codes for malignant lesions are assigned according to:
   a. the size (diameter) of the lesion.
   b. the extent of the malignancy and associate metastases.
   c. the type of repair used to correct the defect caused by the excision.
   d. the measurement of the skin margins taken, plus the size of lesion.

4. The purpose of CPT is to provide a _____ _____ for communication among physicians, patients and third party payers.
   a. reimbursement system
   b. uniform language
   c. data collection and information management system
   d. HCPCS system

5. When coding fracture care in CPT, open treatment is defined as
   a. a fracture site that is surgically opened for repair.
   b. attempted reduction of a fracture with anesthesia.
   c. treatment using cast materials or other immobilizers.
   d. placement of fixation wires across the fracture site for reduction.

6. What component is not included in the CPT definition of a surgical package?
   a. preoperative care
   b. postoperative care
   c. local anesthetic
   d. complications from procedures performed

7. The key component(s) driving the level of Evaluation and Management codes is/are the
   a. face-to-face time of the visit by the physician.
   b. nature of the presenting problem and risk of complications.
   c. history, examination, and medical decision-making necessary.
   d. risk of morbidity and mortality affecting the complexity of diagnosis.

8. If a pathologist or radiologist must review the results of a diagnostic test that is represented by a global or complete CPT code, the code selected must be modified with modifier _____ to indicate that only the professional component of the procedure is being reported.
   a. -76
   b. -26
   c. -25
   d. -77

9. The technical component of a CPT code represents which of the following?
   a. the services of the specialist required to interpret the results
   b. the resources required to perform the test
   c. the facility portion of the procedure including the technician and the equipment
   d. the use of modifiers for enhanced reporting to third party payers

10. Modifiers indicate which of the following?
    a. A physician assistant cannot perform a service or procedure.
    b. A service or procedure was cancelled by the patient.
    c. A service or procedure was somehow changed without the original description being altered.
    d. Additional fees will be charged for a service or procedure.

11. Guidelines for CPT are found
    a. within the index and appendices.
    b. at the beginning of sections and/or subsections.
    c. within the code descriptions.
    d. within HCFA program manuals and health plan contracts.

12. Biopsy codes are arranged in CPT
    a. by extent of tissue removed.
    b. within the same subsection of the Surgery section.
    c. according to pathologic diagnosis.
    d. by anatomic location of the lesion or cyst.

13. Wound closures are classified in CPT by
    a. length of each single laceration.
    b. extent of repair of underlying structures such as nerves and blood vessels.
    c. location, size, and tissue involvement.
    d. type of sutures used.

14. An excision results in a wound that requires intermediate closure. How should this be reported?
    a. Code both the excision and the intermediate closure.
    b. Code the excision only, since repair is included in that code.
    c. Code only the intermediate repair, since lesion excision is included in repair codes.
    d. Code the excision with modifier -22 appended to reflect unusual circumstances.

15. Which type of health care provider would *not* use CPT codes for reporting of services?
    a. physical therapists
    b. pharmacists
    c. nurse midwives
    d. clinical psychologists

16. Most hearing tests are binaural. If a patient has only one ear tested during an encounter, how should the service be coded?
    a. Code the hearing test with modifier -52 for a reduced service.
    b. Use codes for those tests with "unilateral" in the description.
    c. Use the HCPCS modifiers RT or LT for "right" or "left."
    d. Use modifier -22 for unusual service.

17. If a CPT code description says "list separately in addition," "report in addition to," "is to be added as an additional procedure," or "each additional," which of the following rules is true?
    a. Reimbursement for this procedure will be less than if it were coded by itself.
    b. Modifier -51 does not apply to this code, and the code with this description is coded without any other codes.
    c. Modifier -51 does not apply to this code, and the additional services are always reported with another code.
    d. The additional services are integral to the primary procedure code, so modifier -59 will be appended to these codes to obtain extra reimbursement from health plans.

18. How is ligation of vessels in an open wound coded?
    a. by the appropriate code in the Cardiovascular section of CPT
    b. by referencing "suture, vessels" in the CPT index
    c. by selection of complex repair codes, then by size of the wound
    d. No code is needed for this procedure since ligation is included in the repair codes.

19. Which statement is true about the APC system of reimbursement?
    a. APCs are used for hospital outpatient surgery.
    b. APCs are "driven" by CPT codes.
    c. APCs will be used for all outpatient reimbursement systems after January 1, 2000.
    d. APCs will be useful to physicians for data collection.

20. Lysis of adhesions with abdominal surgery requires careful coding assessment. Which of the following reflects appropriate coding practice?
    a. An additional code is always added for the lysis of adhesions.
    b. Modifier -59 is assigned to the procedure code for the lysis to show that the procedure was separate from the primary procedure.
    c. No additional code is assigned unless the adhesions were extensive and required additional resources to complete the operation.
    d. The coder maximizes reimbursement for his or her employer by assigning the additional code.

21. Closed fracture treatments represented by CPT codes include which three methods?
    a. without manipulation, without anesthesia, and without reduction
    b. with manipulation, without manipulation, or with or without traction
    c. with traction, without traction, or with manipulation
    d. with or without internal fixation

22. Hospitals are required to report "visits" to HCFA for Medicare patients. Which section of CPT codes is used for this purpose?
    a. codes from the Medicine section of CPT
    b. hospital visit codes
    c. codes from the Evaluation and Management section of CPT
    d. the lowest level procedure code section in CPT

23. A patient was seen in the physician's office Monday morning and the physician advised the patient's family that nursing home placement was recommended to care for advanced senile dementia, posing a danger to the patient and family members. That afternoon the physician admitted the patient to Pleasant View Care Center, but did not see the patient until the next day. Which category(s) of services in CPT should be used to report the physician's services for this patient on Monday?
    a. Nursing Facility Services
    b. Care Plan Oversight Services
    c. Office and Other Outpatient Services, and Nursing Facility Services
    d. Office and Other Outpatient Services

24. If a gastroenterologist performs a flexible sigmoidoscopy examination where two specimens are collected by brushing, what is the correct code?
    a. 45330
    b. 45331
    c. 45378
    d. 45300

25. Code the following procedure: Treatment of a child burned by hot coffee. First degree burns were documented, dressed with Silvadene cream and bandages.
    a. 16020
    b. 16010
    c. 16000
    d. Dressings do not warrant a CPT code.

26. How many codes will be assigned to surgical arthroscopy of the knee with meniscus repair and shaving?
    a. two codes: one for the arthroscope and one for the meniscus repair
    b. one code, since the approach is included in the surgical procedure in CPT
    c. three codes: one for the approach, one for the repair, and one for the shaving of the meniscus
    d. only one code, the arthroscopy of the knee with or without synovial biopsy

Resources

American Medical Association, *Current Procedural Terminology (CPT)*. Chicago: American Medical Association, 1999.

AdminiStar Federal Inc., *National Correct Coding Policy Manual for Part B Carriers*. Indianapolis, IN, 1995.

Federal Register, Vol. 63, No. 173/Tuesday, September 8, 1998/Proposed Rules pp. 47552–47836.

Fordney, Marilyn Takahashi, *Insurance Handbook for the Medical Office*, Fifth Edition. Philadelphia: W.B. Saunders Publishing Co., 1998.

Kirschner, Celeste G., Executive Editor, *CPT Assistant*, Chicago: American Medical Association.

Knaus, Gary M., *Getting Paid for What You Do: Coding for Optimal Reimbursement*. Frederick, MD : Aspen Publishers, 1994.

Kotoski, Gabrielle, M., *CPT Coding Answers for Optimal Physician Payment*. Frederick, MD: Aspen Publishers, 1994.

Nicholas, Toula, *Basic CPT/HCPS Coding*. American Health Information Management Association, 1998.

Spiers, Lynn, Editorial Director, *Code It Right*. Salt Lake City: Medicode, Inc., 1998.

Spiers, Lynn, Editorial Director, *CPT Billing Guide: Medicare Billing and Compliance Handbook*. Salt Lake City: Medicode, Inc., 1998.

St. Anthony Publishing, *St. Anthony's Guide to APC and ASC Groups: A Clinical Coding and Reimbursement Reference for Hospitals and ASCs*. Alexandria, VA: St. Anthony Publishing, Inc., 1998.

St. Anthony Publishing, *St. Anthony's Guide to Evaluation and Management Coding and Documentation*, Third Edition. Alexandria, VA: St. Anthony Publishing, Inc., 1998.

St. Anthony Publishing, *St. Anthony's Medicare Billing Compliance Guide*. Alexandria, VA: St. Anthony Publishing, Inc., 1998.

St. Anthony Publishing, *St. Anthony's Modifiers Made Easy*. Alexandria, VA: St. Anthony Publishing, Inc., 1998.

Index

Answers to Review Exercises

Chapter 1

1. b
2. c
3. a
4. d
5. b

Chapter 2

1. d
2. c
3. b
4. a
5. c

Chapter 3

1. c
2. a
3. b
4. d
5. b

Chapter 4

1. Case Assessment:

Due to space restrictions we do not have a complete case, so it is assumed we will code for the services contained within this documentation only. We can approach the case from a physician perspective, or from a facility or hospital perspective:

Physician Services: We have one date of service represented consisting of a history and physical encounter and a cardiac catheterization service performed by the same physician. At the time of case assessment, the coder performing an analysis of this case should ask the following questions:

1. Are there any services provided before the H&P rendered on 12/4 or following the cardiac cath? When an episode of care is reported, all dates of service surrounding the episode are normally billed together. The documentation should be reviewed for prior consultation services, hospital visits, or subsequent surgery. For hospital services this information is irrelevant.

2. Do I have all the necessary reports? (Not in this sample, since progress notes are not available and it is not known if they proceeded with the attempted PTCA or bypass procedures following the catheterization.) When coding more than one procedure, the procedure with the most value (highest charge, greatest RVU, or most resource intensive) is listed first. Of course it is very important to include all services rendered for coding so the optimal amount of revenue earned is paid and no charges are missed.

Hospital Services: The hospital will only be assigning CPT codes to report the facility services for the cardiac catheterization. Additional codes for other tests such as X-rays and laboratory tests will likely be assigned automatically by the Charge Master program. In some hospitals, coders do not assign the cardiac catheterization and angiography codes in CPT since these are assigned automatically when the procedure is performed.

2. *Overview of Key Reports:*

The H&P is reviewed to establish the appropriate code range and level of service according to CPT or payer-specific guidelines. The physician may report an Evaluation and Management code for the initial hospital visit in the range of 99221-99223. Because this patient has a comprehensive history, a comprehensive examination is documented, and the medical decision making is of high complexity, the highest level of code may be assigned. To confirm this, the coder uses the current documentation guidelines for Evaluation and Management services. This is why it is important to note the details within the documentation of the H&P. Also, inclusion of all pertinent diagnoses helps to substantiate the higher levels of medical decision making.

Note that the medication list includes Glucophage. The physician should be queried to confirm an additional diagnosis of Type II Diabetes, which likely is affecting patient management and should be coded as a secondary diagnosis.

The presence of a diagnostic procedure is identified by the presence of the cardiac catheterization report.

3. *Data from Clinical Reports:*

The coder looks here for the details for coding the procedure, either for the physician's service or facility portion. It is noted that this is a left cardiac catheterization (93510) without mention of cutdown or ventricular puncture, which would lead to different code assignment. Also found is the selective angiography of the right and left coronaries (93545) and left ventricular cine angiography (93543).

4. *Evaluation and Exclusion:*

During this phase of the CODER method, the codes selected for the procedure are examined to see if one code is a component of any of the others. According to the National Correct Coding Initiative edits, these procedures are appropriately reported together, since they are by nature separate from each other. The introduction, positioning, and repositioning of the cathethers are included in the cardiac catheterization code, so they would not be separately reported.

5. *Review, Refinement and Reimbursement Impact:*

For physician reporting, the coder may consider the reimbursement effect of code selection according to payer guidelines. If Mrs. Patient were a Medicare patient the services would be paid according to a fee schedule amount based on a Resource Based Relative Value System (RBRVS). The coder then determines if the resulting payment is reasonable and/or appropriate for the service. If the resulting reimbursement seems incorrect for the service documented, the coder should review other resources to assure all appropriate codes have been assigned.

In the proposed APC system for Medicare reimbursement, the hospital would assign the codes for the procedure, which would result in the APC group assignment 958 (Left Heart Catheterization, Retrograde, From the Brachial Artery, Axillary Artery or Femoral Artery, percutaneous) which is eligible for an expected payment of $1,381.03. The injection for angiography codes are "packaged" with the cardiac catheterization, so it does not result in additional reimbursement for the hospital.

Chapter 5

1. The number 5 statement "The services performed in the locations that qualify for coding in this protocol" is not addressed.

2. Your response should include wording similar to the following:
"Emergency Room Services as those rendered by Emergency Department assigned physicians in the Emergency Department of ABC Hospital. Emergency Room codes are not assigned to clinic patients, hospital observation status patients, or hospital outpatients receiving ancillary services only."

Chapter 6

1. c
2. d
3. a
4. c
5. d

Chapter 7

Surgical Coding Exercises

1. 21325
2. 00402, P1 or 19318 for payers who do not accept anesthesia codes
3. 44156
4. 58150
5. 59409
6. 54150
7. 52332
8. 51715
9. 15000 + 15100
10. 33517, 33533
11. 52332
12. 30520, 31255
13. 31629
14. 17000, 17003, 17003
15. 29880
16. 29892
17. 67805
18. 66983
19. 69631
20. 54057

Radiology Coding Exercises

1. c
2. b
3. d
4. b
5. c

Pathology and Laboratory Coding Exercises

1. c
2. a
3. b
4. d
5. b

Medicine Coding Exercises

1. c
2. d
3. c
4. a
5. b
6. a
7. c
8. b
9. c
10. a

Chapter 8

1. b
2. d
3. d
4. b
5. a

Appendix

1. c
2. c
3. a
4. b
5. a
6. d
7. c
8. b
9. c
10. d
11. b
12. d
13. c
14. a
15. b
16. a
17. c
18. d
19. b
20. c
21. b
22. c
23. d
24. a
25. c
26. b